Radiology of the Abdomen and Pelvis

A succinct account of various routinely experienced pathologies and suitable images has been presented as approximately 162 case studies. The cases are structured into thematic chapters with an integrated approach to basic learning. Each case study follows a similar format with a brief clinical presentation, relevant imaging findings, discussion with differential diagnosis, management, and suggested readings. This book focuses on the pointwise description of cases routinely encountered in abdominopelvic imaging that help students, trainees, and radiologists to write certificate examinations.

Key Features:

- Presents chapters in the form of case studies, along with a brief illustrative description of normal anatomy and abnormal findings.

- Uses image-based quizzes for easy comprehension for trainees, residents, and practicing radiologists.

- Incorporates pivotal cases from the hepatobiliary, pancreatic, genitourinary, and gastrointestinal systems in a single book.

Dr. Swati Goyal is an Associate Professor of Radiodiagnosis at GMC Bhopal and has been keenly involved in academics, research, and public health work. She has three international books to her credit: two as an author—*Neuroradiology: A Case-Based Guide* and *Essentials of Abdomino-Pelvic Sonography* published by CRC Press, Taylor & Francis Group—and one as an editor, *Clinical Sonography: A Practical Guide SAE*—published by Wolters Kluwers. She is also the author of a non-academic book addressing public health issues pertaining to lifestyle ailments, *What a Non-medico Must Know: The Quintessential Guide to Family Health and Wellness*. She was awarded a PhD in Medicine for her work on machine learning in medical imaging, and her papers on the topic have been accepted at multiple prestigious international conferences. She is a coordinator of a national AI committee, IRIA and AI course coordinator, ICRI. She is also a recipient of the President's Appreciation Award by the Indian Radiology and Imaging Association (IRIA) 2022.

Radiology of the Abdomen and Pelvis
A Case-Based Guide

Swati Goyal

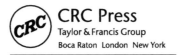

CRC Press
Taylor & Francis Group
Boca Raton London New York

CRC Press is an imprint of the
Taylor & Francis Group, an **informa** business

Front cover image: Shuttersctock

First edition published 2025
by CRC Press
2385 NW Executive Center Drive, Suite 320, Boca Raton FL 33431

and by CRC Press
4 Park Square, Milton Park, Abingdon, Oxon, OX14 4RN

CRC Press is an imprint of Taylor & Francis Group, LLC

Library of Congress Cataloging-in-Publication Data
Names: Goyal, Swati, author.
Title: Radiology of the abdomen and pelvis : a case-based guide / Swati Goyal.
Description: First edition. | Boca Raton : CRC Press, 2024. |
Includes bibliographical references and index. | Summary: "A succinct account of various routinely experienced pathologies and suitable images has been enlisted as approximately 150 case studies. The cases are structured into thematic chapters with an integrated approach to basic learning. Each case study follows a similar format with a brief clinical presentation, relevant imaging findings, discussion with differential diagnosis, management, and suggested readings. The book focuses on the pointwise description of cases routinely encountered in abdominopelvic imaging that help students, trainees and radiologists to write certificate examinations"—Provided by publisher.
Identifiers: LCCN 2024022079 (print) | LCCN 2024022080 (ebook) |
ISBN 9781032588780 (hardback) | ISBN 9781032587745 (paperback) | ISBN 9781003452034 (ebook)
Subjects: MESH: Abdomen—diagnostic imaging | Pelvis—diagnostic imaging |
Abdomen—pathology | Pelvis—pathology | Radiology—methods | Case Reports
Classification: LCC RD540 (print) | LCC RD540 (ebook) | NLM WI 141 |
DDC 617.5/5075—dc23/eng/20240628
LC record available at https://lccn.loc.gov/2024022079
LC ebook record available at https://lccn.loc.gov/2024022080

ISBN: 9781032588780 (hbk)
ISBN: 9781032587745 (pbk)
ISBN: 9781003452034 (ebk)

DOI: 10.1201/9781003452034

Typeset in Palatino
by codeMantra

Dedication

This work is dedicated to my remarkable parents for ingraining the virtues of diligence and perseverance in me. With deepest gratitude, I acknowledge the profound impact of their hard work and love on my professional and personal growth.

Contents

Preface

CT and MRI have revolutionized diagnostic imaging since their inception in the early 1970s and have become the backbone of medical imaging. As we are broadening our horizons in the arena of CT/MRI applications, so must the erudition of technologists occupied in this field.

My enthusiasm for case-based learning blossomed during my radiology residency. Not only are the cases brief, engaging, and entertaining, but they also reflect the challenges that radiologists encounter on a daily basis. This book offers a few cherry-picked cases with a concise account of approximately 162 routinely experienced pathologies and suitable images of patients presenting in myriad ways. The cases are structured into thematic chapters, rendering an integrated approach to basic learning. Each case study has been drafted, commencing with a brief clinical history, pertinent imaging findings, discussion with differential diagnosis, management, and suggested readings for every chapter.

This book is formulated as a succinct teaching guide for the core exam, American Board of Radiology—radiology residents, general practitioners, and CT and MRI technicians. The text will be helpful to other general physicians, gastroenterologists, nephrologists, and urologists interested in medical imaging, even though this book is primarily intended for trainee radiologists, surgeons, and CT/MRI technicians.

This book is organized into nine thematic chapters, followed by the image-based quiz.

Chapters 1 and 2 include cases involving the hepatobiliary, spleen, pancreas, and gastrointestinal systems. They also cover embryology, anatomy, and normal and pathological findings with differential diagnoses and relevant images, typically seen during routine practice. Topics such as congenital, infective, inflammatory, traumatic, benign, and malignant neoplastic lesions of the liver, spleen, biliary system, pancreas, and gastrointestinal tract have been compendiously described.

Chapters 3–6 elucidate embryology and normal anatomy of the genitourinary system, including the kidney, ureter, bladder, male and female genital system, and adrenal glands, with routinely seen case studies in a few well-chosen words. Along with a brief explanation of normal anatomy, Chapters 7 and 8 also comprise cases of the aorta, inferior vena cava, diaphragm, peritoneum, retroperitoneum, and anterior abdominal wall lesions.

The imaging findings of abdominal tuberculosis, which can involve the ileocecum, liver, spleen, mesentery, peritoneum, retroperitoneum, and genitourinary tract, are described in Chapter 9. The image-based quiz of 30 questions at the end of this book serves as a rapid review tool.

Appropriate training and expertise are required, along with theoretical knowledge of cases for reporting. This book is an adjunct to standard textbooks and is not intended to substitute them. This book focuses on pointwise description of cases routinely encountered in abdominopelvic imaging and helps in writing certificate examinations such as the core exam of ABR (American Board of Radiology), RITE (Residency In-service Training Exam) of the American Academy of Radiology, CAQ (Certificate of Additional Qualification) exam, ARRT (American Registry of Radiology Technicians), BSc (Bachelors of Science) in medical imaging, and ARMRIT (American Registry of Magnetic Resonance Imaging Technologists).

Bolstered by nearly 220 high-resolution images obtained with state-of-the-art scanning technology, this essential enchiridion is promptly accessible to interpret both CT and MRI images of the hepato-biliary-pancreatic region, gastrointestinal tract, genitourinary region, vascular branches, and peritoneal region. It includes valuable contextual material, such as case studies commonly encountered in clinical practice, besides normal anatomy, that equips the reader with the challenges of the clinical setting. It can be used as an expedited reference amid a busy clinical day.

This book aims to provide a consolidated resource for technologists to acquire the knowledge imperative for excellent patient care.

Acknowledgments

Transforming an idea and conceptualizing it into a book is as arduous as it sounds; the experience is both internally challenging and gratifying. I would wholeheartedly like to thank the individuals who contributed to the realization of this achievement.

Authoring a fourth technical publication proves to be more challenging than anticipated, although it also yields greater satisfaction than initially envisioned. This remarkable accomplishment would not have been possible without my husband, Dr. Sanjay Goyal, MD Paediatrics, IAS, MPH (JHU), who has been my rock throughout my career, providing invaluable guidance and encouragement throughout my professional journey. Much love and thanks to my children Prisha and Rushank for their unwavering support and understanding during the countless hours of research and writing. Their encouragement has been a constant source of motivation. I am deeply grateful to my in-laws for their unwavering emotional support and encouragement.

I am deeply indebted to my esteemed mentors, Dr. OP Tiwari and Dr. Rajesh Malik, whose profound influence has motivated me to pursue an academic path.

A task of this size could not be effectuated without the unwavering support provided by our head of department, Dr. Lovely Kaushal—many thanks to her insightful academic perspective and affirmative influences.

I am grateful to Dr. RP Kaushal for his professional guidance and support. I would also like to extend a profound thanks to my seniors and colleagues, Dr. Vijay Verma, Dr. Poornima Maravi, Dr. Ankit Shah, Dr. Mallika Singhai, Dr. Bhagat, and Dr. Rambharat, for their generous support. Heartfelt thanks to Dr. Sahil Gupta and Dr. Shimanku Maheshwari for their enthusiastic support during this venture.

Many thanks to Dr. Anita Uikey (SR) and my postgraduate students from GMCH Bhopal—Dr. Shubham Aggarwal, Dr. Nayan, Dr. Rakesh, Dr. Pallavi, Dr. Malay (JR-3), Dr. Shubham Lekhwani, Dr. Nitin, Dr. Kunika, Dr. Lavanya, Dr. Arjun Jat, and Dr. Alok Gupta (JR-2) for collecting cases as well as for their technical support.

Special thanks to Dr. Abhinav Sharma, Dr. Arushi Kaushal Bang, Dr. Aastha Dixit, Dr. Bhavana Saraf, Dr. Neha Chandel, Dr. Prakhar Jain, Dr. Sanchi Gulati, and Dr. Shubham Rai, from SAIMS, Indore, for collecting cases.

I would like to acknowledge and appreciate all the authors and editors whose publications, including books, journals, and websites. I have gone through this since my medical residency days. Their invaluable contributions have provided access to cutting-edge research, imaging facilities, and resources that played an indispensable role in the creation of this book.

Immense thanks to Miranda Bromage, publisher, Taylor & Francis, CRC Press, Daina Habdankaite, and Shivangi Pramanik, Senior Commissioning Editor-Medical, and her editorial assistant Lavanya Sharma and Hudson Greig, who green-lighted this book and stayed patient throughout its lengthy gestation. Earnest thanks to Ms. Ramya, the project manager and her team, especially the skilled graphic design team of codeMantra. Writing a comprehensive technical book on abdominopelvic radiology is a collaborative effort involving many individuals' contributions and support. I am expressing my deepest gratitude to the following who have substantially contributed to the content of this endeavor.

Dr. Mahesh K Mittal, MBBS, MD
Professor and Head, Radiodiagnosis,
Subharti Medical College, Meerut
(45 images)

Dr. Pramod Sakhi, MBBS, MD
Professor, Radiodiagnosis
Sri Aurobindo Institute of Medical Sciences,
   Indore
(15 images & 5 case studies)

Dr. Bhavin Zumkhawala, MD
Consultant Radiologist
Ahmedabad
(1 image & case study)

Dr. Lovely Kaushal, MBBS, MD
Professor & Head, Radiodiagnosis
Gandhi Medical College, Bhopal
(65 images)

Dr. Prateek S. Gehlot, MBBS, MD
Associate Professor, Radiodiagnosis
R.D. Gardi Medical College, Ujjain (M.P.)
(15 images)

Dr. Vipul Virabhai Solanki
Associate Professor, Radiodiagnosis
Government Medical College, Bhavnagar
   (Gujarat)
(10 images)

Dr. Digish Vaghela, MD
Associate Professor, Radiodiagnosis
B.J. Medical College Ahmedabad
(6 images and 6 case studies)

Dr. Supriya Chadgal
HoD Radiodiagnosis
Shatabdi Hospital, Govandi, Mumbai
(7 images)

Dr. Poornima Maravi, MBBS, MD
Associate Professor, Radiodiagnosis
GMCH Bhopal
(4 images)

Dr. Sana Mirchia Varma, MBBS, MD
Senior Resident
Chhindwara Institute of Medical Sciences,
    Chhindwara (M.P.)
(10 case studies)

Dr. Bhagat Yadav
Assistant Professor, Radiodiagnosis
Gandhi Medical College, Bhopal
(2 images)

Dr. Arunima, MD, DNB
Consultant Radiologist
Sanya Diagnostic Center, Bhopal
(2 case studies)

Dr. Rambharat
Senior Resident
GMCH Bhopal
(2 images)

Dr. Anjali Singal
Associate Professor, Anatomy
AIIMS, Bathinda
(Anatomy & Embryology)

Dr. Ratnesh Jain, MBBS, MD
Assistant Professor, Radiodiagnosis
GRMC, Gwalior (MP)
(13 line diagrams).

Dr. Mallika Singhai, MBBS, MD
Assistant Professor, Radiodiagnosis
Gandhi Medical College, Bhopal
(2 images)

Dr. Ankit Shah
Assistant Professor, Radiodiagnosis
Gandhi Medical College, Bhopal
(4 images and 2 case studies)

Dr. Bhagyashree, MD, DNB, EDiR
Fellow, Neuroradiology
University of Cincinnati, Ohio
(25 images)

Dr. Kavan Parikh
Senior Resident
BJ Medical College, Ahmedabad
(4 images and 3 case studies)

Dr. Sarath AS, JR-3
GMCH Bhopal
(Anatomy & Embryology)

List of Abbreviations

AA	Abdominal aorta
AI	Artificial intelligence
AML	Angiomyolipoma
a/w	associated with
CBD	Common bile duct
CDUS	Color Doppler ultrasound
CHD	Common hepatic duct
CKD	Chronic kidney disease
CMD	Corticomedullary differentiation
CSI	Chemical shift imaging
CTA	CT Angiography
D/Ds	Differential diagnosis
DCBE	Double-contrast barium enema
DIE	Deep infiltrating endometriosis
DWI	Diffusion-weighted imaging
EAS	external anal sphincter
EPN	Emphysematous pyelonephritis
ERCP	Endoscopic retrograde cholangiopancreatography
ESR	Erythrocyte sedimentation rate
FNAC	Fine needle aspiration cytology
GNETs	Gastric neuroendocrine tumors
GB	Gallbladder
GC	Greater curvature
GEJ	Gastro-esophageal junction
GIT	Gastrointestinal tract
GOO	Gastric outlet obstruction
HCC	Hepatocellular carcinoma
HU	Hounsfield Units
IAS	Internal anal sphincter
IC	Ileocaecal
IHBR	Intrahepatic biliary radicals
IMA	Inferior mesenteric artery
IVC	Inferior vena cava
k/c/o	known case of
LC	Lesser curvature
LRV	Left renal vein
MPD	Main pancreatic duct
PaNETs	Pancreatic neuroendocrine tumors
PCS	Pelvicalyceal system
PD	Pancreatic Duct
PDG	Paraduodenal groove
PTC	Percutaneous transhepatic cholangiogram
PUJ	Pelvi-ureteric junction
RCC	Renal cell carcinoma
RLQ	Right lower quadrant
ROI	Region of interest
RUQ	Right upper quadrant
SA	Surface Area
SAAG	Serum ascitic albumin gradient
SBO	Small bowel obstruction
SI	Signal intensity
SMA	Superior mesenteric artery
s/o	suggestive of
T1WI	T1-weighted images
T2WI	T2-weighted images
TB	Tuberculosis
TRUS	Transrectal ultrasonography

UGI	Upper Gastrointestinal
UTI	Urinary tract infection
VCUG	Voiding cystourethrogram
VUJ	Vesicouretric junction
XGP	Xanthogranulomatous pyelonephritis
XGC	Xanthogranulomatous cholecystitis

1 Hepatobiliary-Lieno-Pancreatic System

INTRODUCTION

Embryology

The liver develops from an endodermal hepatic bud during the fourth week of intrauterine life. The hepatic bud divides to form a larger pars hepatica, which forms the liver, and a smaller pars cystica, which forms the gall bladder (GB) and cystic duct (Figure 1.1).

The pancreas develops from ventral and dorsal pancreatic buds, which are also endodermal in origin. Before the midgut rotation, the ventral bud lies anteriorly, and the dorsal bud lies posteriorly to the duodenum. With the rotation, the ventral bud and the bile duct come to the right, and the dorsal bud comes to the left of the duodenum. Due to the differential growth of the gut wall, the ventral and dorsal pancreatic buds move closer (star) to each other and finally fuse to form a single mass in the seventh intrauterine week.

Two ventral and one dorsal pancreatic buds appear during the fifth week of pregnancy. Next, the ventral buds fuse. The duodenum enlarges by the seventh week, stimulating the conjoined ventral bud to rotate posteriorly and merge with the dorsal bud. The ventral bud forms the inferior part of the uncinate process, the pancreatic head, and the body and tail by the dorsal bud. The fusion of the ducts of ventral and dorsal buds forms the main pancreatic duct (MPD) (Figure 1.2).

Anatomy

Liver

The liver is a major organ in the RUQ of the abdominal cavity and is encapsulated by Glisson's capsule. It is almost entirely covered by visceral peritoneum except in the gallbladder fossa, IVC fossa, and the bare area. It is divided into functional regions called lobules, further divided into smaller units called sinusoids. The porta hepatis is a transverse fissure in the liver hilum that contains the portal vein, hepatic artery, and right and left hepatic ducts.

With its dual blood supply, the liver gets 75% from the portal vein and 25% from the hepatic arteries. The three hepatic veins draining into IVC constitute the venous drainage. The joining of splenic and superior mesenteric veins, posterior to the pancreatic neck, forms the portal vein—the vein then courses superiorly, posterior to the common bile duct and hepatic artery.

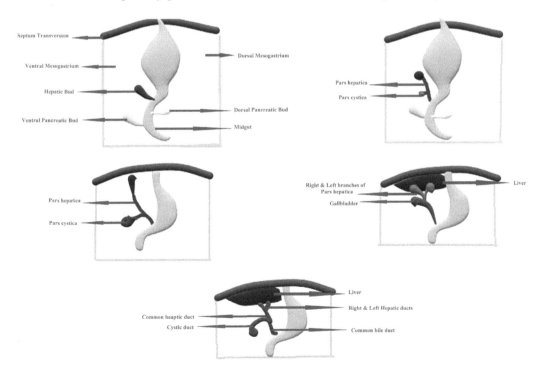

Figure 1.1 Embryology of the liver.

DOI: 10.1201/9781003452034-1

1

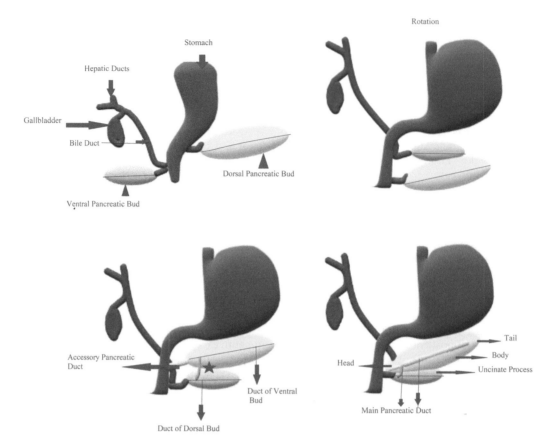

Figure 1.2 Embryology of the hepatobiliary pancreatic system.

Segmental Anatomy

The Couinaud classification describes the liver's functional anatomy, which divides it into eight independent segments. Each segment has its blood supply, biliary drainage, and lymphatic drainage. The liver is divided into the right and left lobes by the middle hepatic vein plane running from the left of the IVC to the left of the gallbladder fossa.

The right lobe is bifurcated into anterior and posterior sectors by the plane of the right hepatic vein that lies in the right intersegmental fissure.

The anterior sector includes segments V and VIII, and the posterior segments include VI and VII. The horizontal portal vein plane divides them into the superior (VII and VIII) and the inferior segments (V and VI).

The plane of the left hepatic vein and the falciform ligament splits the left lobe into medial and lateral sectors. A horizontal portal plane further divides the liver divides each section of the liver into superior and inferior segments. The left lateral sector includes segment II, which lies above, and segment III, below the portal plane. Segment IV lies between the middle and left hepatic veins, and this left medial sector incorporates segment IVa above and segment IVb below the portal plane.

Segment I/caudate lobe is bounded anteromedially by the fissure for ligamentum venosum. It is described as a separate entity, receiving blood supply from the right and left portal veins, drained directly into the IVC (Figure 1.3).

Gallbladder

The GB is a pear-shaped reservoir of bile and lies on the inferior surface of the liver. The average adult gallbladder is 3–4 cm wide and 8–10 cm long. GB comprises the fundus, body, infundibulum, and neck. The cystic duct combines the common hepatic duct (CHD) and forms the common bile duct (CBD). The cystic artery supplies the gallbladder, which is drained into the portal vein by the cystic veins.

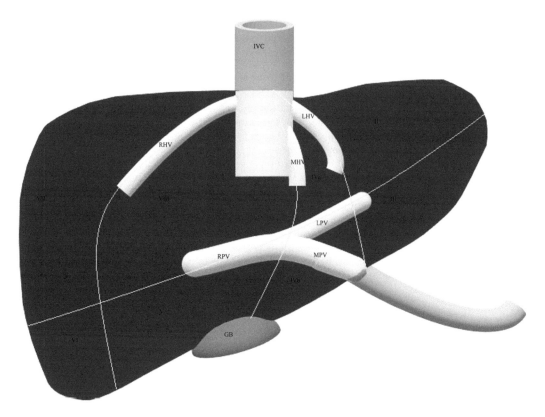

Figure 1.3   The segmental anatomy of the liver.

Pancreas

The pancreas is a retroperitoneal organ comprising the head, uncinate process, neck, body, and tail. A network of pancreatic ducts extending throughout the gland secretes pancreatic juice.

The superior and inferior pancreaticoduodenal arteries feed the head of the pancreas. The dorsal pancreatic artery, greater pancreatic artery (arteria pancreatica magna), and transverse pancreatic artery are splenic branches supplying the neck, body, and tail. Numerous tiny veins drain blood to the splenic hilum. The inferior pancreaticoduodenal vein empties into the superior mesenteric vein, while the superior pancreaticoduodenal vein drains into the portal vein.

Biliary Tree

The portal venous supply of the liver parallels the biliary anatomy. The bilateral hepatic ducts drain the right and left lobes of the liver, respectively. The anterior right hepatic duct (ARHD) drains segments V and VIII in the anterior liver, and the posterior right hepatic duct (PRHD) drains segments VI and VII in the posterior liver. The ducts draining segments II, III, and IV combine to form the left hepatic duct (LHD). The portal triad comprises the bile ducts, hepatic artery, and portal vein branches. At the porta hepatis, the right and LHDs merge to form CHD. The gall-bladder's cystic duct joins the CHD to create the CBD with a standard diameter of less than 6 mm. CBD enters the pancreatic head and combines the MPD at the major duodenal papilla to form the ampulla of Vater, where a ring-shaped smooth muscle band called the sphincter of Oddi encircles the MPD and the distal end of the CBD.

RECIST Criteria

Response to treatment to evaluate tumor burden, preferably by CECT/MRI/PET, is assessed by RECIST (Response evaluation criteria in solid tumors) criteria.

The lesions are categorized as measurable (target lesions such as sum of longest diameter (SLD) of tumor >10 mm, short axis diameter of lymph node >15 mm, soft tissue component of bony metastasis, etc.) and non-measurable lesions (ascites, pleural effusion, lymphangitis, miliary metastasis, small metastasis in liver, lungs, etc.). A follow-up scan is done after at least 1 month of therapy to determine the response in the form of complete/partial regression of the lesions, stable disease without any change, or progression in the lesion size or appearance of new lesions.

Liver Imaging Reporting and Data System

Liver Imaging Reporting and Data System (LI-RADS) CT/MRI diagnostic algorithm provides a structured approach for a radiologist's classification of liver lesions to reduce inter-reader inconsistency and, thus, produce more precise diagnoses. It is mainly applicable to patients with chronic liver disease/cirrhosis, the most significant risk factor for liver cancer, and not meant for patients under 18 years with vascular etiologies of cirrhosis.

The LR1 to LR5 categorization system is based on specific imaging findings of the lesion and correlates to the degree of risk for malignancy. It ranges from LR1 (definitely benign: cysts, hemangiomas, focal fat sparing/deposition, or any lesion which regresses spontaneously), LR2 (probably benign: T1 hyperintense and T2 hypointense siderotic nodules and perfusion abnormalities of parenchyma such as transient hepatic attenuation differences), LR3 (intermediate, < 10 mm), LR4 (probably malignant, 10–19 mm), LR5 (definitely malignant, > 19 mm), noncategorizable (NC) nodules, LR-TIV (tumor-in-vein), and LR-M (malignancies other than HCC). The suspicious nodules from categories 3 to 5 are categorized based on arterial phase hyperenhancement, washout, and capsule enhancement characteristics.

Normal Variants

- Reidel's lobe of the liver

  A tongue-like projection of the anterior edge of the right lobe of the liver extending downwards. No displacement of the kidney or other intraperitoneal organs differentiates it from hepatomegaly.

- Beaver-tailed liver (a sliver of the liver) (Figure 1.4)

  The elongated left lobe of the liver extends laterally and wraps around the spleen. It is prone to injury in blunt abdominal trauma or may be mistaken as peri splenic hemorrhage or pseudo masses. Color Doppler depicts the normal hepatic and portal vessels.

- Prominent papillary process of the caudate lobe

  Medial projection of the caudate lobe, which can be mistaken for lymphadenopathy or a pancreatic body mass.

- Phrygian gallbladder

  Folding of GB fundus

- Lobulated spleen

  Lobulations of the spleen usually disappear before birth but may sometimes persist.

- Accessory spleen

  Congenital defect due to the severe lobulation of the spleen and nipping off of splenic tissue, as well as the failure of embryonic splenic buds to fuse inside the dorsal mesogastrium. Typically, a splenic artery branch supplies the accessory tissue, which drains into splenic veins. Attenuation and enhancement are similar to that of the spleen.

- Splenic clefts

  The notches or clefts are the remnants of the groove and may mimic laceration.

- Upside-down spleen

  An abnormal splenic rotation results in the superior hilum, and the convex border is medial and adjacent to the left kidney.

- Lobulated pancreas

  Extension of the pancreatic parenchyma anteriorly, posteriorly, or horizontally simulating the pseudo masses.

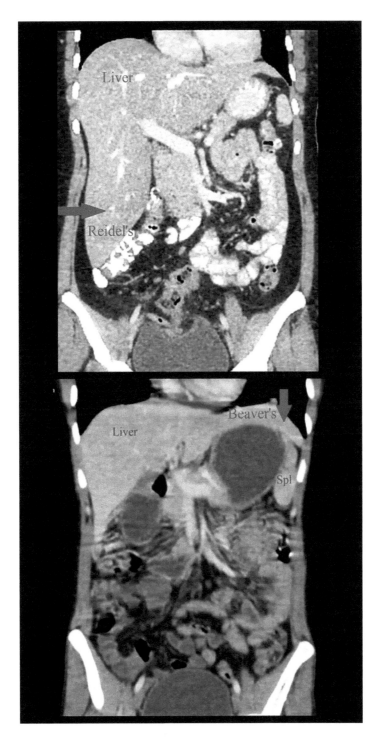

Figure 1.4 Reidel's lobe and beaver-tailed liver, the normal variants.

- Arterial and biliary tract variations

  Accessory and replaced hepatic arteries

  Accessory bile ducts, variations in cystic duct insertion, right posterior hepatic duct draining into the left hepatic duct, etc.

PATHOLOGIES

LIVER

Case 1 Pyogenic Liver Abscess

A 33-year-old male presented with moderate fever, anorexia, mild hyperbilirubinemia, and RUQ pain for 5 days (Figure 1.5).

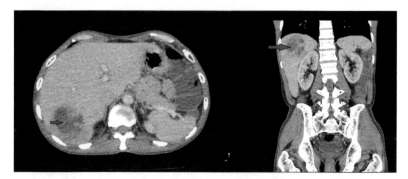

Figure 1.5 Hepatomegaly with an ill-defined peripherally enhancing hypodense lesion involving segment VII of the liver.

Discussion

Focal collection of necrotic inflammatory tissue in the liver parenchyma due to various infective agents (parasitic, bacterial, and fungal). The most common location is the right lobe. Other nonspecific findings include pleural effusion, basal atelectasis, and raised hemidiaphragm. Free intra-peritoneal rupture, hepatic or portal vein thrombosis, biliary compression, and communications may occur in a few complicated cases. It is challenging to differentiate either of these etiologies on imaging and can be confirmed by serology and microbiology.

Differential Diagnosis (Table 1.1)

Other differentials include:

- Infected hydatid cyst

- Necrotic metastases

- Cystic HCC

- Biliary cystadenoma

Table 1.1: Different Infective Etiologies of Liver Abscess

Bacterial	Fungal	Parasitic (Amoebic)
Multiple	Multiple	Single
Staph aureus, *E. Coli*, anaerobes, TB	Candida, Histoplasma, CMV	Entamoeba Histolytica
Portal or biliary route	Hematogeneous route	Oro-fecal route
Fluid density multilocular lesion with internal echoes, irregular shaggy walls, and peripheral rim enhancement (target sign) associated with the cluster of similar small coalescing lesions near the large lesion. May contain air foci within Central pus is hypointense on T1WI, hyperintense on T2WI, and shows restricted diffusion due to the high viscosity of pus on DWI. The inner and outer layers of the wall appear hypo- and hyperintense on T2WI, respectively.	Multiple, diffusely scattered, hypodense areas (1–2 cm in diameter). These lesions may involve both liver and spleen Sonography depicts a "Wheel within wheel" appearance with a centrally necrotic, hypoechoic area of fungal debris, surrounded by a hyperechoic and hypoechoic rim of inflammatory cells and fibrosis, respectively. Common in immunocompromised patients and may be associated with lymphoma. Differentials include liver metastases, miliary TB, lymphoma, septic emboli, and sarcoidosis.	Large, relatively smooth, and well-defined, unilocular, hypodense lesions near the liver periphery (posterior segment). Characteristic anchovy sauce pus may be aspirated. May be a/w traveler's diarrhea. Colon involvement (colonic wall thickening) is found in a few cases.

Management

- Mild cases respond to medical therapy.

- Moderate to severe cases may require image-guided percutaneous drainage.

Case 2 Hydatid Cyst

A 25-year-old patient presents with vague abdominal discomfort and a routine checkup (Figures 1.6 and 1.7).

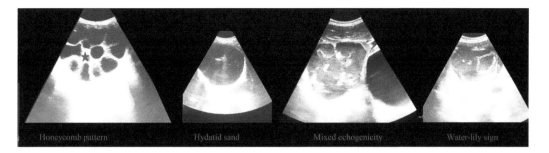

Figure 1.6 Sonography depiction of the characteristic appearance of cysts enclosed within a cyst-honeycomb (*) pattern seen in a hydatid cyst, an anechoic cyst with hydatid sand, a hydatid matrix of mixed echogenicity containing scolices, membranes of broken daughter vesicles, hydatid sand serpentine linear structures within the cyst—Water Lily sign.

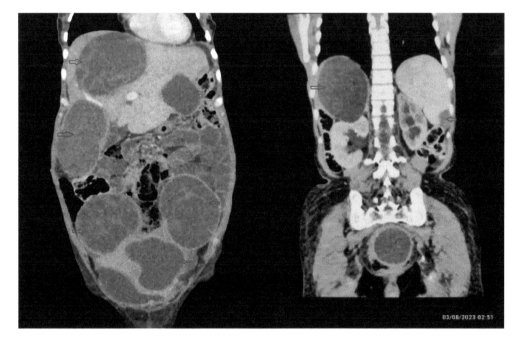

Figure 1.7 CT scan showing the honeycomb pattern in a hydatid cyst with the multiple septae representing the walls of daughter cysts. CT scan shows hydatid cysts of varying sizes and patterns in the liver, spleen, and peritoneal cavity.

Discussion

Hydatid disease, commonly caused by *Echinococcus granulosus*, is a parasitic infection with dogs as an intermediate host. These can occur anywhere in the body, with the liver being the most common site, followed by the lungs and other parts of the body. Type IV cysts are complicated ones with rupture (contained, communicating, or direct) or superinfection.

An enzyme-linked immunosorbent assay (ELISA) is used to confirm the diagnosis.
Cyst structure (Table 1.2)
Classification (Table 1.3)
Imaging findings on various modalities (Table 1.4)

Table 1.2: Cyst Structure

Pericyst	Host's Inflammatory Response to Parasite
Ectocyst	Passage of nutrients
Germinal layer	Daughter vesicles are produced
Daughter cysts	Daughter vesicles detached from the germinal layer

Table 1.3: Cyst Classification

Type I - CE1	Unilocular cyst with thin rim enhancement
Type II - CE3	Water lily sign—Ruptured cyst with floating membranes
Type III - CE2	Spoke-wheel/Honeycomb pattern—Multiple small daughter cysts within the mother cyst +/−wall calcification
Type IV - CE4	Echogenic matrix (solid appearing lesion—ball of wool sign)
Type V - CE5	Densely calcified cyst (with posterior acoustic shadowing on sonography and hypointensity on MRI

Table 1.4: Radiological Findings of Hydatid Cyst on Various Imaging Modalities

Sonography	Double-line sign—a hypoechoic layer separates two echogenic lines of the cyst wall. (c.f. simple cysts, cystic tumors, pseudocysts, or metastases)
	Snowstorm sign—Multiple echogenic scolices (sand) fall to the dependent portion of the cyst, noted by repositioning the patient
	Heterogeneously echogenic lesions with collapsed membranes (serpentine structures) within the matrix
	"Water lily sign" or "camalote sign"—Ruptured hydatid cysts with floating parasitic membranes in the fluid
	Multiple daughter cysts within parent cyst
	Multiple vesicular cysts within a large cystic lesion
CT scan	Unilocular/multilocular, thin-walled cyst with peripherally located and low-attenuated daughter cysts
	Detects calcification in the cyst wall or septa
	CECT shows internal septal enhancement and no wall enhancement
	Evaluates complications and is efficacious in cases of obesity, excessive bowel gases, abdominal wall deformities, and previous surgery
MRI	The characteristic appearance of a cystic part is a low signal intensity on T1WI, a high signal on T2WI, and a low signal intensity rim on both T1 and T2WIs due to the collagen-rich pericyst layer. Daughter cysts appear hypo to isointense relative to the matrix on T1WI and T2WI. Floating membranes appear as hypointense serpentine structures
	DWI shows restriction in hydatid cysts due to internal viscous contents compared to simple cysts

Hydatid cysts may communicate with the biliary tree or rupture with free spillage into the peritoneal cavity, resulting in peritoneal seeding (hydatidosis). It may result in a contained rupture if the pericyst is intact.

Differential Diagnosis

This type of picture is characteristic of hydatid without any differentials. But simple liver cysts, choledochal cysts (CDCs), Caroli's disease, hemangioendotheliomas, mesenchymal hamartomas, and teratomas may be considered in the differentials of hepatic hydatid. Splenic cystic lesions include epidermoid and dermoid cysts, solitary abscesses, hematomas, cystic hemangiomas, intrasplenic pancreatic pseudocysts, and lymphangiomas. Understanding various imaging presentations of hydatid disease may help decrease diagnostic lag and reduce the risk of fatal consequences.

Management

- Chemotherapy (prior to therapeutic intervention and in inoperable cases)

  PAIR: **P**uncture of the cyst wall, **A**spiration of cyst contents, **I**nstillation, and **R**easpiration of the scolicidal agent, which disrupts the germinal layer of the cyst. Reduces the cyst size. Avoided in ruptured cysts that communicate with the biliary tree/calcified/dead cysts.

- *Surgery*: Gold standard

Case 3 Hepatitis

A 35-year-old male presents with abdominal pain, anorexia, and vomiting for 6–7 days. Laboratory tests confirmed elevated serum bilirubin (direct 7 mg/dL) and increased LFTs (Figure 1.8).

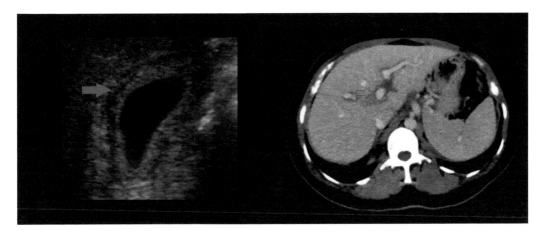

Figure 1.8 The edematous gall bladder wall thickening on sonography and periportal hypoechoic halo on the CECT abdomen.

Discussion

Inflammation of liver parenchyma is due to different types of viral hepatitis. Most patients recover and do not progress to chronic hepatitis. In very few cases, it may progress to fulminant liver failure with abrupt and severe liver dysfunction. Imaging depicts hepatomegaly with the increased brightness of portal vein radicle walls and relatively reduced liver echogenicity, giving a starry sky pattern on sonography. CECT arterial phase depicts periportal hypodensity, inhomogeneous perfusion depending on disease severity, and subsides post-recovery. Transient liver dysfunction due to viral hepatitis is usually associated with ascites and stratified (edematous) gallbladder wall thickening. High T2 signal around the portal system and mild generalized increase in parenchymal signal intensity apart from gradual periportal enhancement may be noted on MRI. Regional lymphadenopathy may be present. Chronic hepatitis shows decreased brightness and number of portal vein radicle walls and overall increased liver echogenicity.

Differentials Diagnosis

- Cholecystitis is a/w localized tenderness and gallstones.
- Autoimmune hepatitis with absent LAP.

Management

Treatment depends on the etiology of acute hepatitis.

Case 4 Cirrhosis with Portal Hypertension

A 51-year-old chronic alcoholic patient presented with RUQ pain, fatigue, and raised LFTs (Figures 1.9–1.11)

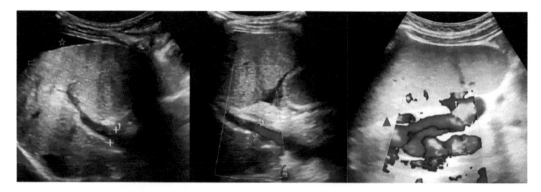

Figure 1.9 Sonography depicts the coarsened echo texture of the liver (open arrow) with irregular margins and mild ascites (star). Narrowing of the portal vein with hepatofugal flow (solid arrow). Moderate splenomegaly (arrowhead) with dilated splenic vein and peri splenic collaterals.

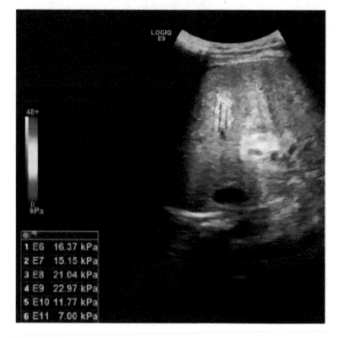

Figure 1.10 Elastography scan reveals 15 kPa elasticity (F4)—cirrhosis. Findings are suggestive of cirrhosis with portal hypertension.

Discussion

Cirrhosis is considered an irreversible, scarred, end-stage liver disease characterized by hepatic fibrosis, distorted liver architecture, and nodularity (Table 1.5).

Sonography findings

- Mild hepatomegaly with heterogeneously coarse and increased liver echogenicity, surface nodularity, widening of fissures, and ascites.

- Hypertrophied caudate lobe and atrophic right lobe of the liver (caudate width: right lobe width>0.65).

- Signs of portal hypertension with dilated portal vein with sluggish flow, mild splenomegaly with dilated splenic vein. In later stages, the liver may shrink.

- Sonoelastography evaluates tissue stiffness and elasticity in kilopascals (kPa), with increasing values correlating to higher stages of fibrosis (Table 1.6).

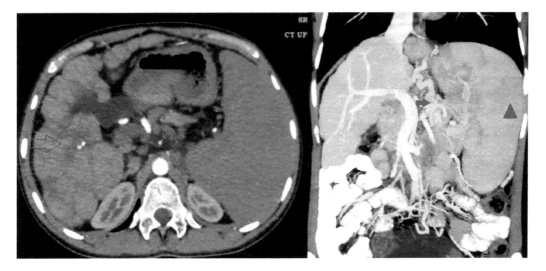

Figure 1.11 CECT abdomen reveals a small cirrhotic liver (open arrow) with multiple nodules leading to irregular contour and moderate splenomegaly (arrowhead). MIP coronal image revealed multiple collaterals (solid arrows) at the perigastric, peri esophageal, and lienorenal regions— Cirrhotic liver with features of portal hypertension.

Table 1.5: Types of Cirrhosis

Type	Micronodular	Macronodular
Nodules size	Uniform involvement of the liver Size<3mm	Irregular involvement with interspersed normal liver tissue Size>3mm
Association	Alcoholic liver disease, hemochromatosis, bile outflow, and hepatic vein obstruction	α-1 antitrypsin deficiency, chronic viral hepatitis, primary biliary cholangitis, Wilson disease

Table 1.6: Liver Stiffness Values

>7–10 kPa	Advanced chronic liver disease and fibrosis
> 12.5 kPa	Cirrhosis
> 21 kPa	Portal hypertension

The METAVIR score (F0: no fibrosis, F1: portal fibrosis without bridging fibrosis, F2: portal fibrosis with few bridging fibrosis, F3: bridging fibrosis with architectural distortion, F4: cirrhosis)

A 6-monthly sonography is recommended to rule out HCC as a complication. Endoscopic gastroduodenoscopy (EGD) is done to screen esophageal varices.

Color Doppler Ultra Sound (CDUS)

- *Hepatic Vein*: Spectral broadening, hepatic vein narrowing, dampening of phasic oscillations in hepatic venous flow.

- *Portal Vein*: Initial dilatation (>1.4 cm diameter) followed by reduction of diameter due to formation of collateral vessels.

- *Hepatic Artery*: High resistive index, but developing a large arteriovenous or arterioportal shunt leads to lower resistance.

CT—In the early stages, the liver may appear normal. With disease progression, cirrhotic liver depicts contour nodularity, changes in volume distribution with an enlarged caudate lobe and left lobe lateral segment, atrophy of the right and left lobe medial segments, widening of the fissures and the porta hepatis, and regenerative nodules.

Spectrum of nodules in cirrhotic liver (Table 1.7)

Table 1.7: **Characteristics of Cirrhotic Nodules**

Types	Diameter	Imaging Findings	Nature
Regenerative nodules (RN) → Multiple	1–5 mm	Distinct margins, non-enhancing (siderotic nodules may appear hyperdense)	Benign
Dysplastic nodules—few can be Low-grade (LGDN) or High-grade (HGDN)	10–15 mm	Vague, early enhancement without washout	Relatively risk depending on grade
Hepatocellular carcinoma (HCC)	> 15–20 mm	Vague, early enhancement with washout	Definite

Two stages of cirrhosis (Table 1.8)

Table 1.8: **Stages of Cirrhosis**

Compensated Cirrhosis	Decompensated Cirrhosis
Early, mild stage	Deteriorated liver dysfunction
Without complications	Complications—Esophageal varices, hepatic encephalopathy, hepatopulmonary syndrome, and hepatorenal syndrome

Differential Diagnosis

1. Siderotic nodules due to iron accumulation

2. Low-grade dysplastic nodules

3. *Small HCCs*—Early arterial enhancement with washout.

4. *Liver metastases*—High T2WI

5. *Pseudo cirrhosis*—Retracted and scarred parenchyma, post-chemotherapy, in patients with hepatic metastasis.

Ultrasound-guided liver biopsy is the gold standard for diagnosis of liver cirrhosis.

Portal Hypertension

It is characterized by an abnormally high-pressure gradient in the portal circulation; the most common cause is extrahepatic portal venous obstruction in children and cirrhosis in adults. Imaging findings include dilated portal vein, portosystemic collaterals, splenomegaly, and ascites. Complications include variceal bleeding, spontaneous bacterial peritonitis, hepatorenal syndrome, and hepatic encephalopathy.

Table 1.9 discusses the normal and abnormal values of portal circulation.

Table 1.9: **Measurements Differentiating Normal Individuals from Patients with Portal Hypertension**

Values	Normal	Portal Hypertension
Portal pressure (mm Hg)	7–10	> 10
Hepatic venous pressure gradient	1–4	> 5 > 10 (varices) > 12 (bleeding, ascites)
Portal vein diameter (mm)	< 13	> 13
Splenic vein diameter (mm)	< 10	> 10
Flow	Hepatopetal with normal undulations	Hepatofugal, monophasic
Congestion index (cm sec) = Cross-sectional area of portal vein/Blood flow in portal vein	< 0.075	> 0.08

Management

- Medical therapy (beta-blockers for varices and diuretics for ascites)
- Interventions for bleeding varices in cirrhotic patients
- TIPSS (Transjugular Intrahepatic PortoSystemic Shunt)
- BRTO (Balloon-occluded Retrograde Transvenous Obliteration)
- Variceal embolization

Case 5 Liver Trauma

A 25-year-old male presented after RTA (Figure 1.12).

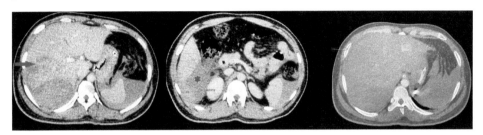

Figure 1.12   CECT abdomen depicts mild hepatomegaly with multiple irregularly linear non-enhancing hypodense tracts in segments V, VI, and VII suggestive of lacerations (solid arrow). Hyperdense subcapsular collection (HU +42) along segments VI & VII of the liver with a maximum depth of 4.1 cm s/o hematoma. No evidence of active contrast extravasation or vascular injury was noted. Linear undisplaced fracture (open arrow) of the anterolateral aspect of the 7th rib. A moderate amount of hyperdense fluid (+34 HU) in the pelvic and peritoneal cavity s/o moderate hemoperitoneum.

Discussion

The liver is among the most frequently injured organs. Initial assessment is done through FAST (Focused Assessment with Sonography for Trauma) to look for fluid/hemorrhagic collection in peritoneal, pleural, and pericardial cavities. CT scan better evaluates injuries, such as lacerations, hematomas, and vascular injuries (pseudoaneurysms, arteriovenous fistula-localized accumulation of vascular contrast which attenuates compared to active bleed, which increases in the delayed phase). It assesses delayed complications such as abscesses, peritonitis, leaks, etc., and guides for further management by interventional techniques. Arterial and portal venous phases are better for delineating vascular complications. Table 1.10 discusses the grades of liver, spleen, and kidney injuries.

Management

Spontaneous healing with conservative treatment.

Surgery for hemodynamically unstable cases.

Table 1.10: Grading of Injury to Liver, Spleen, and Kidney in Trauma Patients

		Liver	Spleen	Kidney
Grade I	Laceration (parenchymal depth); capsular tear	< 1 cm	< 1 cm	No
	Subcapsular hematoma (surface area)	< 10%	< 10%	Present
Grade II	Laceration parenchymal depth	1–3 cm	1–3 cm	< 1 cm (no involvement of collecting system)
	Subcapsular hematoma (SA)	10%–50%	10%–50%	Confined perirenal hematoma
	Intraparenchymal hematoma <10 cm (diameter)	< 10 cm	< 5 cm	

(Continued)

Table 1.10: (Continued) Grading of Injury to Liver, Spleen, and Kidney in Trauma Patients

		Liver	Spleen	Kidney
Grade III	Laceration	>3 cm	>3 cm	> 1 cm (no involvement of collecting system
	Subcapsular hematoma	> 50%	> 50%	
	Intraparenchymal hematoma/rupture	> 10 cm	> 5 cm	
	Vascular injury with active bleed	Confined within liver parenchyma	–	Contained within the perirenal fascia
Grade IV	Laceration (organ involvement)	25%–75% Breaching the liver parenchyma into the peritoneum	With > 25% devascularization of hilar/segmental vessels	Involves collecting system (urinary extravasation) Segmental renal a/v injury with active bleeding extending beyond the perirenal fascia
	Vascular injury with active bleeding		Contained within the splenic capsule	
Grade V	Laceration	>75%	Shattered spleen	Shattered kidney
	Vascular disruption		Active bleeding extending beyond the spleen into the peritoneum	Renal hilar injury (main renal a/v) with active bleeding

Source: Modified from 2.

Case 6 Hemangioma

A 35-year-old male came for routine sonography and further evaluation (Figure 1.13).

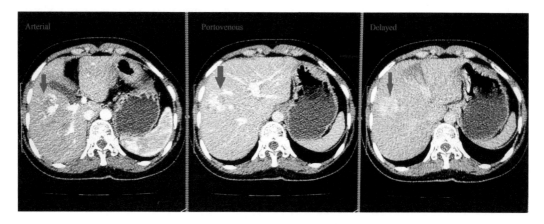

Figure 1.13 Triple-phase CT abdomen depicts a relatively well-defined hypoattenuating lesion in segment V of the liver showing peripheral discontinuous nodular enhancement in the arterial phase, centripetal filling of contrast in the portovenous and delayed phases.

Discussion

Hemangiomas, the most frequent solid liver lesion, are slow-growing and benign and constitute multiple vascular channels lined by single-layered endothelial cells and interspersed thin fibrous stroma. They are usually found incidentally or may present with symptoms related to complications. Types are given in Table 1.11.

Table 1.11: Various Types of Hemangiomas

Small (Capillary Type)	< 2 cm	Homogeneous Enhancement (Flash-Filling)
Typical (cavernous type)	2–10 cm	Progressive centripetal enhancement to uniform filling
Atypical/Giant	> 10 cm	Incomplete filling

14

Differential Diagnosis

Focal fat sparing/deposition, cirrhotic nodules, hemangioendothelioma, metastasis, etc. The rest of the details are discussed in Table 1.12

Table 1.12: Differential Diagnoses for Solid Liver Lesions

	Hemangioma	Hepatic Adenomas	HCC	Fibrolamellar HCC	Hepatic Metastasis (Most Common)	Focal Nodular Hyperplasia (FNH)
Age/gender	Middle-aged females	Young females	Elderly males	Young (<40)	Elderly	-
Common associations	High cardiac output lesions	Obesity, diabetes, OCPs Hemorrhage propensity	a/w cirrhosis, hepatitis B and C virus, smoking, alcoholism, hemochromatosis, aflatoxins Raised alpha-feto protein	Not a/w underlying liver disease. Normal alpha-fetoprotein	-	
Nature	Solitary, well-circumscribed; peripheral nodular enhancement with centripetal fill-in	Solitary, well-defined, pseudo-encapsulated	Focal, multifocal, and diffuse (infiltrative) patterns with ill-defined borders	Solitary, lobulated lesion with central scar (calcifications +)		Lesion with central scar
Location	Subcapsular, posterior right lobe	Subcapsular	Anywhere			
Sonography	Hyperechoic,	Heterogeneously hypoechoic with a few hyperechoic areas due to fat	Heterogeneous appearance depending on the content-fat, calcification, fluid, hemorrhage	Heterogeneous lesion with the central scar, fibrosis, and calcification	Heterogenous or homogeneous depending on the content (calcium, fat, mucin, fluid)	Isoechoic with hyperechoic central scar
Color Doppler	Low flow without spectral broadening due to slow intralesional flow	Variable flow Perilesional sinusoids	High flow with spectral broadening (AV shunting, angiogenesis)	High flow with spectral broadening	Low flow with spectral broadening	High flow with spectral broadening

(Continued)

Table 1.12: (Continued) Differential Diagnoses for Solid Liver Lesions

	Hemangioma	Hepatic Adenomas	HCC	Fibrolamellar HCC	Hepatic Metastasis (Most Common)	Focal Nodular Hyperplasia (FNH)
NECT/MRI	Hypodense/intense; calcifications rare. T1 hypointense and T2 hyperintense	Hyperdense (hemorrhage) Hypodense (fat) Hyperintense on T1-&T2WI	Heterogeneous lesion depending on the intralesional content and shows restricted diffusion	T1 hypointense, T2 hyperintense with a central T2 hypointense scar	Intralesional content can be visualized	Isodense to the liver with a central star-shaped hypodense scar. The scar is hyperintense on T2WI
Enhancement pattern	Peripheral puddling and nodular enhancement on delayed scan (centripetal progression). Shows the same density as the blood pool in all phases	Early arterial enhancement with isodensity on portal venous and delayed phase	Early arterial enhancement with early "washout." Capsule/rim enhancement may be seen in the delayed phase	Delayed enhancement in the central scar. Does not retain hepato-biliary-specific contrast agents No uptake on Tc99m-S colloid (absent Kupffer cells)	Hypervascular metastases show heterogeneous enhancement in the arterial phase and iso-hypodense/intense in the portal and delayed phases, Wash-out in the PV phase	Homogeneously enhancing lesion in the arterial phase and isodense/intense to the normal liver in all other phases. Central scar enhances the delayed phase Retains hepato-biliary-specific contrast agents Uptake on Tc99m-S colloid seen
Complications	Spontaneous rupture, blessing, mass effect, calcifications, hyalinization, and cystic changes	Spontaneous rupture with hemoperitoneum, malignant transformation	Propensity to involve HVs and PV			

Management

Regular follow-up, if stable. Surgery is indicated in complicated cases.

Case 7 Focal Hepatosteatosis

A 55-year-old female on chemotherapy post-surgery for breast carcinoma (Figure 1.14).

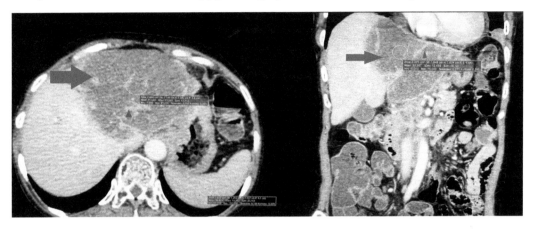

Figure 1.14 CECT abdomens show the geographic area of hypoattenuation (+23 HU) in the left lobe of the liver compared to the rest of the liver parenchyma (+58 HU) with different attenuation.

Discussion

Hepatic steatosis may be a focal/geographical/perivascular or diffuse/multifocal pseudo lesion frequently a/w obesity, insulin resistance, postoperative chemotherapy, alcohol use, metabolic diseases, etc. Common sites for focal steatosis include the porta hepatitis, GB fossa, and medial segment near the falciform ligament.

The lesion is hyperechoic on imaging compared to the adjacent liver parenchyma, spleen, and kidneys. Comparatively, focal fat sparing is hypoechoic to adjacent structures. This geographic type of lesion shows the normal vessels traversing through it without any mass effect.

NCCT shows hypoattenuated lesion (< 40 HU) or attenuation difference of >10 HU (NCCT) and >25 HU (CECT) between the liver and spleen. The lesion depicts T1 hyperintensity with a signal drop on opposed-phase imaging.

Differential Diagnosis

■ Focal hepatosteatosis—hemangioma (characteristic enhancement pattern)

■ Diffuse/multifocal lesion—metastasis (no fat within the lesion)

Management

Conservative

Case 8 Secondary Hemochromatosis

A 24-year-old male with RUQ pain (Figure 1.15).

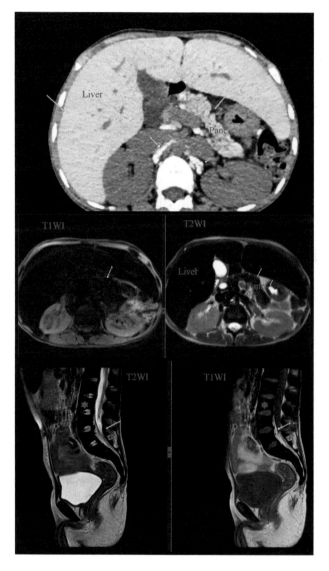

Figure 1.15 Pancreas and liver hyperdense on CT and hypointense on MRI.

Discussion

Hemochromatosis is an iron overload abnormality, with increased iron storage and deposition in various organs such as the liver, spleen, pancreas, etc., leading to organ dysfunction. It could be primary (genetic) or secondary to underlying disease. Secondary hemochromatosis occurs due to frequent transfusions, excessive iron intake, myelodysplasias, etc.

It may present as hyperpigmented (bronze) skin, hepatosplenomegaly, arthritis, heart failure/arrhythmias, hypogonadotropic hypogonadism, diabetes, etc. It may complicate HCC.

Imaging shows homogeneously increased attenuation on NECT with a relatively hypoattenuating portal and hepatic veins in organs with iron deposition. DECT quantifies iron deposition. Vertebral bodies (star), apart from other affected organs such as the liver and pancreas, are hypointense on both T1- and T2WI, with a signal drop on in-phase imaging.

Differentials Diagnosis

- *Hemosiderosis*: Increased iron deposition without organ dysfunction.

- Hyperattenuated liver, spleen, etc. are seen in amiodarone therapy or glycogen storage diseases.

Management

Phlebotomy

Iron chelation therapy

Case 9 Hepatocellular Carcinoma

A 48-year-old male with jaundice (Figure 1.16).

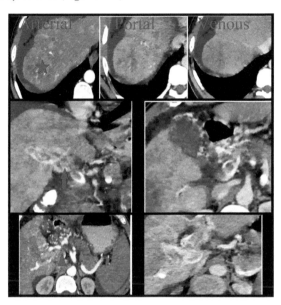

Figure 1.16 Triple-phase CT abdomen depicts cirrhotic liver with a few relatively ill-defined heterogeneously enhancing (early enhancement early washout pattern) lesions (star) scattered in the right lobe of the liver. Dilated portal vein with tumoral thrombus (arrow). Multiple periportal and pericholecystic collaterals (arrowhead). The portal vein shows early enhancement in the arterial phase s/o intrahepatic arterio-porto shunting.

Discussion

HCC, the most frequent primary liver malignancy, is epithelial in origin and presents with jaundice and constitutional symptoms. It could be focal, multicentric, nodular, or infiltrative type with the propensity to invade vascular structures, such as portal vein and hepatic vein, and at risk of thrombosis. Sonography shows hypoechoic or heterogeneous lesions with peripheral hypoechoic rim. The lesion shows early arterial enhancement (neovascularity) with early washout and delayed capsular enhancement. Tumor thrombus shows enhancement compared to bland thrombus. Arterioportal shunting can be seen. HCC metastasizes to the lungs, bones, lymph nodes, and adrenals.

Differentials Diagnosis

This is discussed in Table 1.12. It should also be differentiated from intrahepatic cholangiocarcinoma, lymphoma, granulomatous diseases.

Management

- TACE, RFA, or chemical ablation
- Liver transplantation
- Palliative therapy

Case 10 Liver Metastasis

A 66-year-old male with abdominal discomfort and jaundice (Figure 1.17).

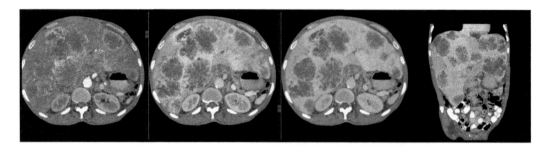

Figure 1.17 CT abdomen depicts hepatomegaly with multiple hypodense heterogeneously enhancing hepatic lesions showing marginal enhancement in the arterial phase followed by subsequent washout.

Discussion

The liver is the most frequent site of metastases due to dual blood supply from the portal and systemic circulation, providing a fertile niche to primary tumors such as GI malignancies, breast, lung, etc. CT is primarily used to assess treatment response. The hyperattenuating rim of the normal liver (due to hemorrhage and coagulative necrosis) surrounding the lesion is included in the treatment process. Hence, the treated lesion appears larger than the original lesion. PET-CT aids in delineating the extent of metastasis. Metastases are usually hypointense on T1WI and hyperintense on T2WI. However, lesions with calcific, fibrous hemorrhagic components are hypointense on T2WI, and melanoma metastases are hyperintense on T1WI (Table 1.13).

Table 1.13: **Types of Metastases**

Hypovascular Metastases	Hypervascular Metastases
Colorectal, lung, stomach cancer, and breast	RCC, melanoma, thyroid, and neuroendocrine tumors Breast (sometimes)
Hypodense (> fluid attenuation), irregular margins, peripheral enhancement	Echogenic on sonography
Best seen during the PV phase	Best seen during the arterial phase

Differential Diagnoses

These are discussed in Table 1.12. Pseudocirrhosis was noted post-chemotherapy in patients with liver metastases from the pancreas, colon, and medullary thyroid cancer.

Management

1. Interventional radiology in the form of radiofrequency ablation, microwave and laser ablation, cryoablation, and alcohol ablation—To debulk tumors and for symptomatic relief.

2. Trans-arterial hepatic chemoembolization (TACE) for locoregional chemotherapy.

BILIARY SYSTEM

Case 11 Retrohepatic Gallbladder

A 24-year-old male with incidental finding (Figure 1.18).

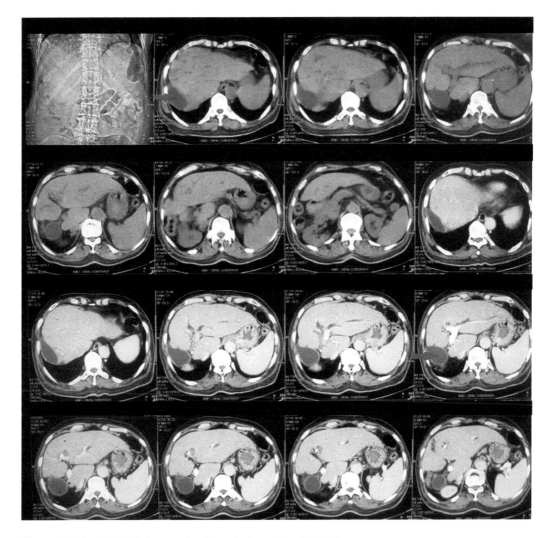

Figure 1.18   CECT abdomen depicts retrohepatic gallbladder.

GB may be positioned ectopically in any location—transversally, under the left hepatic lobe, intrahepatic, and rarely retrohepatic (as in this image).

Congenital anomalies of GB include agenesis, rudimentary, duplicate, multiseptated honeycomb pattern, hourglass shape, Phrygian cap, etc. The wandering GB is due to long mesentery with the risk of torsion.

Case 12 Duplicated Gallbladder

An incidental finding (Figure 1.19).

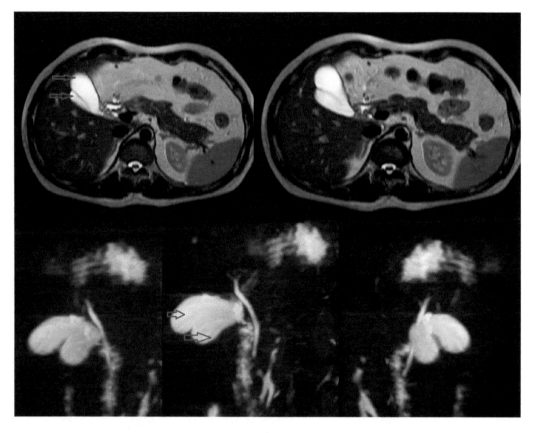

Figure 1.19 MRCP depicts gallbladder duplication.

Discussion

Duplicated gallbladder, an infrequent anomaly, refers to an accessory GB without any propensity for increased malignancy/calculi. It could be

- Partially divided, bilobed GB sharing a single cystic duct
- Fully duplicated GB, with distinct cystic duct and a shared hepatic duct
- Fully duplicated GB, with the common cystic duct connecting to the CHD

Sonography, after fasting, shows the contraction of normal GB and no contraction in duplicated one. MRCP better delineates the anatomy.

Differentials Diagnosis

- Folded GB (stones communicate with all parts)
- Phrygian cap/adenomyomatosis (gallstones may sequester in a compartmentalized part)
- GB diverticulum
- Pericholecystic collection
- Intraperitoneal fibrous Ladd bands (a/w foregut malrotation)

Management

Cholecystectomy in symptomatic cases.

Case 13 Cholelithiasis with Cholecystitis

A 42-year-old obese female presented with RUQ pain, vomiting, and fever (Figure 1.20a).

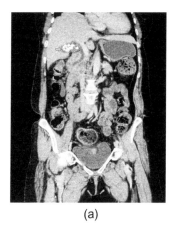

(a)

Figure 1.20a CECT abdomen depicts multiple stones in the gallbladder with associated wall thickening and duct dilatation.

Discussion

Acute cholecystitis is an acute inflammatory thickening of the GB wall with or without obstruction from cholelithiasis. Gallstones may occur due to impaired contractility and can be cholesterol type (10% with >50% cholesterol), pigmented type (saturated with unconjugated bilirubin and could be black due to chronic hemolysis and brown due to parasitic/bacterial infections), and mixed type (80%).

Sonography

- Highly echogenic gallstones with posterior acoustic shadowing and mobility on the patient's repositioning.

- Sonographic Murphy's sign is maximum tenderness over the distended gallbladder with a sonography probe.

- Gallbladder wall thickening (>3 mm)

- Overdistended gallbladder (>4 cm)

- Pericholecystic fluid collection

CT depicts calcified stones as echogenic, cholesterol stones as hypodense, and most of the variety as isodense to bile and challenging to identify. CT scan is used to determine the extra-biliary extent of the disease and evaluate for complications apart from discerning mucosal hyperenhancement and pericholecystic fat stranding. Gallstones appear as signal voids on T2WI MRI/MRCP (Figure 1.20b).

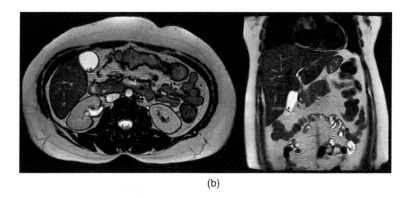

(b)

Figure 1.20b T2WI depicts hypointense round stones showing signal void.

Complications of cholecystitis are given in Table 1.14.

Table 1.14: **Complications of Cholecystitis**

Gangrenous cholecystitis	Mural necrosis of GB with a high risk of perforation resulting in sloughed intraluminal membranes and focal defects in GB mucosa
Emphysematous cholecystitis	Etio-Gas-forming organisms such as *E. coli* Common in diabetics. Gas is seen as reverberation artifacts on sonography and air density foci on CT scans
Mirizzi's syndrome	Cholecystitis+Biliary obstruction Gallstones obstructing the cystic duct/GB neck cause extrinsic compression or erosion of CBD/CHD, resulting in cholecystoduodenal fistula
Pericholecystic abscess	Peripherally enhancing heterogeneously cystic/loculated collections near GB and extending into the adjacent liver parenchyma
GB hemorrhage	Echogenic material intraluminally due to vessel wall destruction
Vascular	PV thrombosis, cystic artery pseudoaneurysm

Management

Cholecystectomy is the treatment of choice for uncomplicated acute cholecystitis with cholelithiasis.

Case 14 Choledocholithiasis

A 30-year-old female with jaundice and abdominal pain (Figure 1.21).

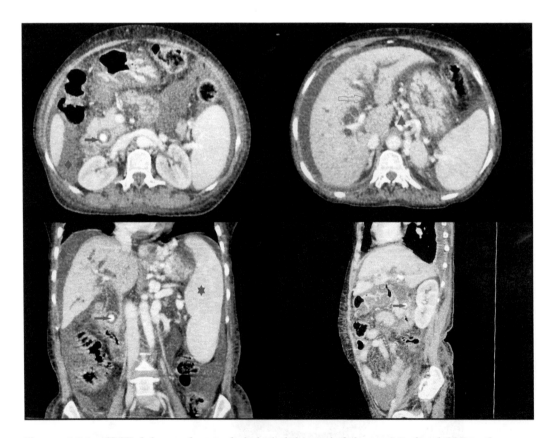

Figure 1.21   CECT abdomen depicts choledocholithiasis (solid arrow) in distal CBD in the pancreatic head with upstream bilateral central and peripheral IHBR dilatation (open arrow). Multiple dilated and tortuous collaterals (arrowhead), gross ascites (diamond), and moderate splenomegaly (star) in this patient with portal hypertension.

Discussion

Choledochocolithiais, CBD calculi, usually a/w multiple small gallstones, can be primary (de novo calculi formation/bile precipitation due to bile stasis and infection; cholesterol/black pigment stones) or secondary (migration of GB stones to CBD; brown pigment calcium bilirubinate stones). The patient may be asymptomatic or may present with biliary colic, jaundice, and a/w cholangitis/pancreatitis.

Sonography depicts echogenic calculi with posterior acoustic shadowing accompanied by proximal ductal dilatation. CT shows calculi as central hyperdensity surrounded by hypodense bile or ampullary soft tissue representing target/crescent sign with abrupt termination of the duct, dilated duct. CECT shows enhancement of a long segment of the bile duct due to associated cholangitis. ERCP shows filling defects and is both a diagnostic and therapeutic option for stone retrieval, sphincterotomy, stent placement, stricture dilatation, tissue sampling, etc., though a/w high risk of complications such as cholangitis, hemorrhage, pancreatitis, etc. MRCP shows stones as hypointense filling defects with hyperintense bile in CBD.

Pitfalls

- Bile precipitation in bizarre forms, such as elongated stones, may misdirect the diagnosis.
- CBD diameter increases post-cholecystectomy and with age; this should be considered during evaluation.
- The most distal part of CBD, coursing through the pancreatic head, should be assessed on sonography with transverse orientation.

Differential Diagnosis

- Filling defects such as air bubbles, ascariasis.
- Surgical clips, vascular calcifications, and partial volume averaging artifacts due to bowel gas.
- Flow voids/susceptibility artifacts on MRCP.
- Malignant causes of CBD obstruction.

Management

Endoscopic sphincterotomy with stone retrieval
Laparoscopic surgery +/– percutaneous biliary drainage depending on the complications.

Case 15 Embolized Biliary Leak

A 52-year-old female patient with post-laparoscopic cholecystectomy status (post-op day-2) and ERCP-guided CBD stenting (plastic stent) presented with sepsis and laparoscopic site bile soaking (Figure 1.22).

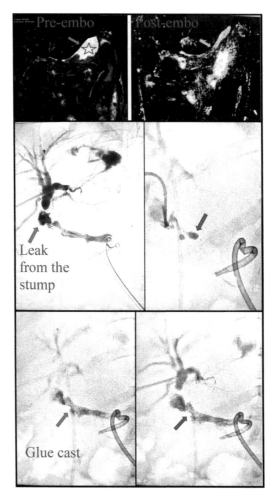

Figure 1.22 MRCP depicting biliary leak to the pocket of collection (blue arrow) from the right anterior sectoral duct without any significant dilatation of IHBRs or CBD. Post-procedure glue embolization shows a collapsed pocket of collection (yellow arrow) and obscured leakage tract. Percutaneous transhepatic cholangiogram depicts a biliary leak from the cystic duct stump (blue arrow). Vividol-glue (2:1) via cobra catheter embolized the leak and the tract (red arrow).

Discussion

Bile leak may occur frequently from cystic duct stump or due to injury to the biliary tree after laparoscopic cholecystectomy or trauma in a few cases. It usually presents as abdominal pain and continuous biliary leakage through the drain.

ERCP and cholangiogram are used for diagnosis. Endoscopic management constituting sphincterotomy and stent placement is used. But embolizing agents, such as vascular coils, micropledgets, NBCA (n-butyl cyanoacrylate), glue, metallic coils, etc., have been used in a few cases.

Case 16 Xanthogranulomatous Cholecystitis

A 70-year-old female presented with abdominal discomfort (Figure 1.23).

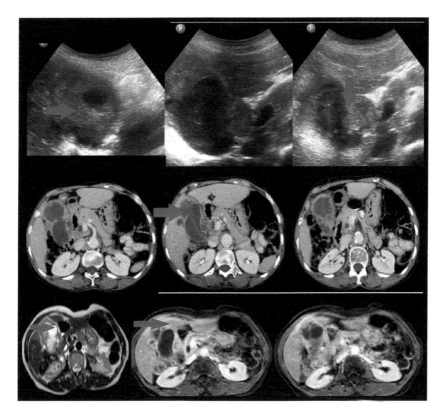

Figure 1.23 Sonography reveals diffuse GB wall thickening with echogenic sludge and tiny calculi entrapped within. CT/MRI reveals diffuse GB wall thickening with heterogeneous enhancement and restricted diffusion.

Discussion

Xanthogranulomatous cholecystitis (XGC) is a rare inflammatory ailment of GB, frequent in elderly females >60. The patient presents with RUQ pain, vomiting, palpable mass, positive Murphy's sign, and obstructive jaundice.

   Imaging reveals diffuse/focal GB wall thickening, intramural hypoechoic/dense nodules, gallstones, loss of fat plane due to adjacent liver infiltration, and heterogeneous contrast enhancement. It may be complicated with abscesses, perforations, and fistulas. Sonography-guided FNAC shows necrotic debris, polymorphs, and foamy histiocytes, confirming the diagnosis. Globally thickened gallbladder wall circumscribing hypoechoic/hypoattenuating/very high T2 signal intensity nodules; continuous mucosal enhancement; absence of intrahepatic bile duct dilation, significant LAP, and of macroscopic hepatic invasion differentiate it from GB malignancy.

Differentials Diagnosis

- GB malignancy
- Chronic perforated cholecystitis
- Cholangitis with periductal infiltration

Management

Cholecystectomy

Case 17 Gallbladder Perforation

A 49-year-old male with acute abdominal pain (Figure 1.24).

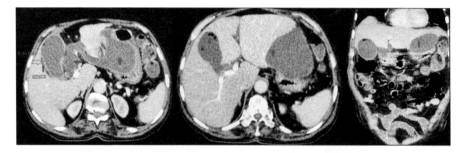

Figure 1.24 CECT abdomen depicts large thin-walled peripherally enhancing hypoattenuating loculated fluid collection (solid arrow) in the pericholecystic region, subhepatic space, lesser sac, and perigastric regions causing liver scalloping. The collection communicates to the fundus and body of GB with a focal defect (open arrow) in the wall and is a/w multiple coarse air foci (arrowhead) in the non-dependent location.

Discussion

Gall bladder perforation (GBP), fundus being the common site, is an infrequent complication of acute cholecystitis, more common in male patients with immunosuppression and co-morbidities such as diabetes and is common with acalculous cholecystitis than calculus cholecystitis. It results in high morbidity and mortality, mandating early management.

GBP can be associated with generalized peritonitis, focal pericholecystic collection, cholecysto-enteric, and cholecysto-biliary fistula. Though sonography is better for delineating gallstones, CT is better for detecting GB complications. Distended GB with an edematous wall is suggestive of impending perforation. Focal wall defect, intramural/luminal air, hemorrhage, sloughed membranes, and pericholecystic collection/abscess/fat stranding may indicate a perforation. If the perforation is not contained, it may result in free air and peritonitis.

Management

Early diagnosis and surgical intervention.

Case 18 Intrahepatic Cholangiocarcinoma with Liver Metastasis

A 64-year-old male came with complaints of abdominal pain and weight loss (Figure 1.25a, b).

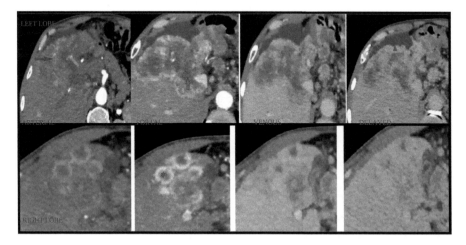

Figure 1.25a Triple-phase CT depicts a large ill-defined lobulated intrahepatic mass (solid arrow) with peripheral continuous arterial phase enhancement and centripetal filling on subsequent venous and delayed phases. Localized left lobe atrophy with capsular retraction (arrowhead), biliary dilatation (open arrow), enhancing lymphadenopathy, and ascites noted—Infiltrating ICC. The right lobe of the liver revealed multiple well-defined, smoothly marginated peripheral enhancing lesions on the arterial and portal phase, along with washout on the delayed phase, suggestive of liver metastasis.

Discussion

Cholangiocarcinomas are adenocarcinomas from biliary tree epithelial lining with poor prognosis, and incidence is less frequent than HCC and GB carcinomas. The patient presents with painless jaundice, anorexia, weight loss, and high alkaline phosphatase, CA-19-9, and gamma-glutamyl transpeptidase. Choledocholithiasis, CDCs, clonorchiasis, primary sclerosing cholangitis, etc., are well-defined risk factors.

CT helps discern tumor extent, biliary dilatation, vascular relationships, lymphadenopathy, and regional and distant spread. The lesion is irregular, hypodense on NCCT, hypointense on T1WI, and hyperintense on T2WI, with gradual centripetal enhancement and intense enhancement on delayed scans, depending on the fibrosis. MRCP assesses longitudinal tumor extent for preoperative biliary mapping. ERCP/PTC has diagnostic and therapeutic options, depicts stricture or filling defects, characterizes anatomy, samples for brush cytology, and plans resectability.

Classification depends on the location (Table 1.15).

Table 1.15: **Types of Cholangiocarcinomas**

Intrahepatic	Extrahepatic Type
Peripheral—distal to the bifurcation of left/right hepatic ducts	Perihilar type (large ducts)
Klatskin's/hilar type arising from the bifurcation of CHD	Distal type (smaller ducts)

Classification of intrahepatic cholangiocarcinoma (ICC) depending on macroscopic growth pattern (Table 1.16).

Table 1.16: **Varying Types of Cholangiocarcinomas**

Mass-forming exophytic type	Mass-type	Distinct liver mass a/w satellite nodules, IHBR dilatation, vascular invasion, capsular retraction. PV obliteration results in segmental atrophy	HCC, liver abscess, metastasis
Periductal infiltrative type	Stricture type	Irregularly thickened tumor along the bile duct wall with proximal biliary dilatation	Benign stricture Periportal/periductal lymphangitic metastasis
Intraductal polypoid type	Mass-type	Enhancing intraductal mass within localized ductal dilatation	Stones within bile ducts Metastatic invasion

Differential Diagnosis

- *Hepatic Abscess:* Thick enhancing wall with cystic necrosis. Regular follow-up scans are required.

- *HCC:* Strong late arterial phase enhancement with rapid washout; usually a/w tumor thrombus.

- *Liver Metastasis:* Central necrosis may be noted.

Management

- Interventional radiology, such as liver ablation, TACE, TARE, etc., or surgery for localized disease.

- Palliative therapy with biliary drainage, via PTBD or EBD, to relieve obstruction and improve patient care.

Another 44-year-old male patient with hilar cholangiocarcinoma presented with jaundice (Figure 1.25b).

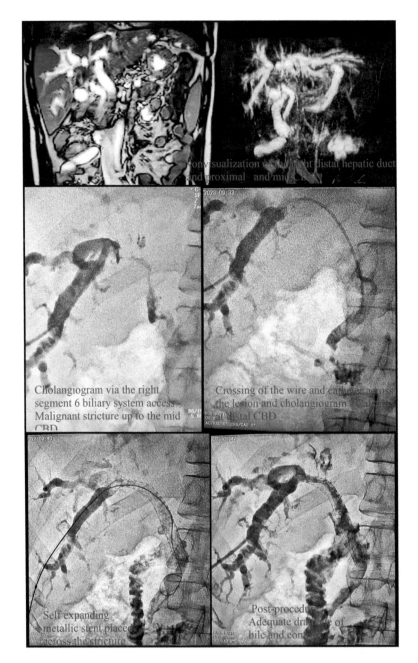

Figure 1.25b MRCP suggested mid-CBD cholelithiasis and near-complete mass infiltration into proximal CBD and right hepatic duct with IHBR dilatation. Cholangiogram via percutaneous biliary access confirmed the diagnosis and extent of the lesion. Hydrophilic wire and catheters were used to cross the lesion, followed by placing the self-expanding metallic stent (8 * 80 mm) across the malignant stricture up to the distal CBD. Adequate bile drainage on the post-stenting cholangiogram.

Case 19 Intraductal Cholangiocarcinoma (Distal Cholangiocarcinoma)

A 51-year-old female with weight loss and anorexia (Figure 1.26).

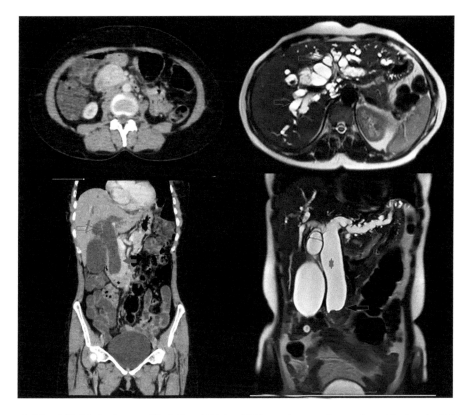

Figure 1.26 MRCP depicts an ill-defined T1 iso, T2 hypointense intra-ductal lesion (solid arrow) with lobulated margins involving distal CBD in the region of ampulla of Vater causing its abrupt termination with upstream gross dilatation of CBD (star), CHD and bilobar central and peripheral IHBR (open arrow).

The details of cholangiocarcinoma have been discussed in the last case.

Differential Diagnosis

Carcinoma of the ampulla of Vater, pancreas, duodenum, and metastasis.

Case 20 Gallbladder Carcinoma

A 50-year-old female presented with RUQ pain and weight loss (Figure 1.27).

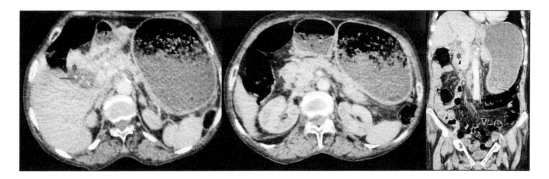

Figure 1.27 CECT abdomen depicts hyperdense calculi (arrow) heterogeneously enhancing asymmetrical thickening (star) involving GB fundus, body, and neck, infiltrating (arrowhead) adjacent liver parenchyma, duodenum, distal stomach antropyloric region, and pancreatic head with fat stranding and proximal dilatation of the stomach.

Discussion

Carcinoma GB is one of the frequent malignancies involving the biliary tract, primarily epithelial in origin, with adenocarcinomas being the most frequent type. It is common in elderly females with cholelithiasis, chronic cholecystitis, and a history of smoking. Patients are initially asymptomatic; advanced cases present with anorexia, weight loss, pain, and jaundice.

On imaging, lesions present as a localized/generalized irregular wall thickening, localized/fungating/polypoidal intraluminal mass, or a large solid lesion with associated cholelithiasis, replacing the GB fossa and infiltrating adjacent structures. Sonography depicts the lesion as an ill-defined, heterogeneously hypoechoic lesion with hyperechoic calcific gallstones. CECT reveals heterogeneously enhancing lesion with interspersed areas of necrosis and calcific foci. It is pivotal to discern the origin of the lesion to narrow down the differential diagnosis. Features suggesting advanced or aggressive malignancy include IHBR dilatation, infiltration of adjacent structures, lymphadenopathy, liver, and distant metastasis. MRI shows heterogeneously enhancing lesion hypo-to isointense on T1WI and hyperintense on T2WI. MRCP delineates the features suggesting advanced disease.

Differential Diagnosis

1. Xanthogranulomatous cholecystitis (with intramural fat nodules)

2. Tumefactive sludge giving pseudotumor appearance (repeat the study)

3. Sloughed mucosa from gangrenous cholecystitis

4. Benign polyps (small size with no heterogeneous enhancement and no interval growth)

5. GB hematomas

6. Perforated cholecystitis (acute pain)

7. Peri cholecystic abscess (toxic clinical presentation of the patient)

8. GB metastasis (look for melanoma, RCC, etc.)

9. HCC/cholangiocarcinoma/duodenal/pancreatic carcinomas or other malignancies invading the GB (essential to discern the origin of the lesion).

Management

Surgical excision in early stages. Advanced cases with infiltration and metastasis require palliative treatment.

SPLEEN

Case 21 Splenic Abscess

A 58-year-old male presented with LUQ pain, fever, and anorexia (Figure 1.28).

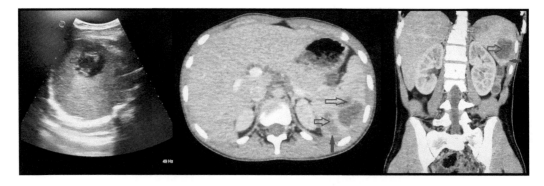

Figure 1.28 USG abdomen shows a solitary well-defined hypoechoic lesion with some internal echoes and septations. CECT abdomen multiseptated, peripherally enhancing hypodense lesions (open arrows) at the mid-lower pole of the spleen. Thinning of splenic parenchyma with a small breach posteriorly leading to subcapsular collection (solid arrows).

Discussion

Splenic abscesses, necrotic collections, are rare owing to the rich reticuloendothelial system of the spleen. It is common in immunocompromised patients. The lesions can be solitary or multiple.

Sonography shows a hypoechoic lesion with internal echoes, fluid levels, and septae of varying thickness. Intralesional gas may cause dirt shadowing in a few cases. CECT shows a hypodense necrotic lesion with peripheral enhancement and enhancing septa.

MRI shows heterogeneously mixed intensity lesions, usually intermediate on T1WI and high on T2WI, due to fluid and proteinaceous content, peripheral enhancement, and restricted diffusion on DWI.

Differential Diagnosis

- Abscesses

  - Pyogenic (due to staphylococcus and streptococcus)

  - Fungal abscess (microabscesses due to candidiasis, aspergillus, etc.)

  - Tuberculosis (irregular miliary pattern or coalescent micronodules)

- Splenic true cysts or post-traumatic pseudocysts

- Hydatid cyst

- Hematomas

- Infarct

- Lymphoma, leukemia, and metastasis

Management

- Medical therapy with intravenous antibiotics

- Sonography—guided percutaneous puncture and drainage

- Splenectomy in refractory cases.

Case 22 Heterotaxy with Polysplenia

A 24-year-old asymptomatic female (Figure 1.29).

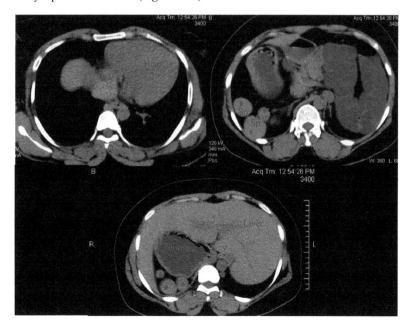

Figure 1.29 CT abdomen depicting transverse liver, multiple splenenculi, intestinal malrotation with right-sided stomach and left-sided bowel loops, and anomalous IVC.

Discussion

Heterotaxy syndrome (situs ambiguus), anomalous left/right position of visceral organs as discussed in the table. Isomerism is a/w midline/transverse liver, intestinal malrotation, and variable location of the stomach (Table 1.17).

Table 1.17: **Various Types of Situs**

Solitus	Normal Orientation of Organs and Vessels in the Body
Inversus	Mirror image of normal
Ambiguus	Visceral malposition and dysmorphism

See Table 1.18.

Table 1.18: **Types of Isomerism**

	Left Isomerism	Right Isomerism
Spleen	Polysplenia syndrome (multiple splenules without a parent spleen)	Asplenia syndrome (abnormal immune status)
Vascular	Azygous/hemiazygous continuation of IVC Preduodenal portal vein, if present, may produce pressure symptoms on the duodenum and bile duct	Severe cyanotic heart disease
Bronchi origin with respect to pulmonary artery	Hyparterial (inferior)	Eparterial (superior)
Lungs	Bilobed	Trilobed
Bilateral atria type	Left	Right
Prognosis	Better	Poor

Diagnosis should be made using chest X-ray, echocardiography, abdominal sonography, and CECT abdomen.

Management

Depends on the malformations and severity of disease.

Case 23 Heterotaxy with Asplenia

An eight-year-old male child presented with cough and breathlessness (Figures 1.30 and 1.31).

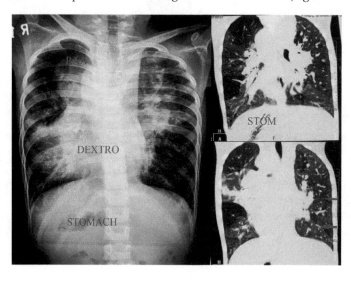

Figure 1.30 CXR and CT chest depicts dextrocardia with right-sided aortic arch, bilateral trilobed lungs, and bilateral infiltrates.

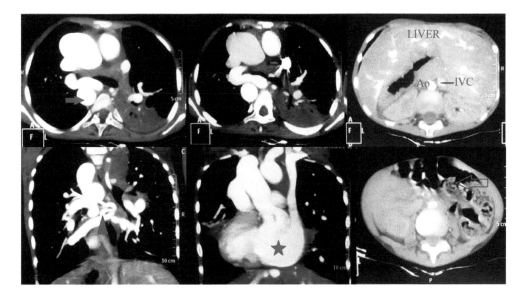

Figure 1.31 CECT abdomen depicts dextrocardia with RAA, single ventricle, ASD, dilated & tortuous abdominal aorta, transverse liver, absent spleen, left-sided aorta and IVC, and gut non-rotation.

Details of this case are discussed in the last case.

Management

Depends on the associated cardiac diseases and malformations.

Case 24 Splenic Trauma

A 25-year-old male with trauma (Figure 1.32).

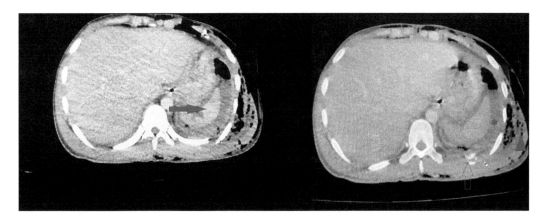

Figure 1.32 CECT abdomen shows a non-enhancing irregularly branched hypodense tract (solid arrow) in the upper pole of the spleen (laceration). Multiple air foci in the peritoneal cavity (pneumoperitoneum), in the subcutaneous and deep intramuscular planes—subcutaneous emphysema (arrowhead), perisplenic hemoperitoneum (star), and fractured left rib (open arrow).

Discussion

Spleen, the most commonly injured solid organ after blunt trauma, presents with LUQ pain, referred pain to the shoulder, and hypotensive shock. Splenic clefts, the normal variant with persistent smooth lobulations, are differentiated due to the absence of hemoperitoneum, hematomas, and other injuries.

The solid organ injuries are discussed in Table 1.10.

PANCREAS

Case 25 Acute Pancreatitis

A 50-year-old female presented with acute pain abdomen (Figure 1.33a).

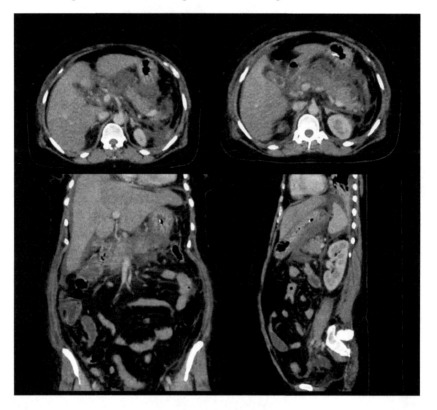

Figure 1.33a CECT abdomen depicts a diffusely bulky pancreas with fuzzy margins and peripancreatic fat stranding. Hepatomegaly with mild pleural effusion and mild ascites.

Discussion

Pancreatitis is inflammation of the pancreatic parenchyma, with gallstones and alcoholism being the most common causes. The other risk factors include hypertriglyceridemia, trauma, ERCP, certain medications, infections, and structural and congenital anomalies.

Patients present with acute epigastric pain radiating to the back and raised serum amylase and lipase levels. Severe cases may be a/w flank ecchymosis (Grey Turner's sign) or periumbilical hematoma (Cullen's sign) (Tables 1.19 and 1.20).

Table 1.19: Phases of Pancreatitis

Early Phase	Late Phase
Occurs within the first week of disease onset. May resolve or progress to late phase	Initiates within the second week. Lasts for weeks to months
Early inflammation due to peripancreatic edema and ischemia	Local and systemic complications

Table 1.20: **Types of Pancreatitis**

Acute Interstitial Edematous Pancreatitis	Acute Necrotizing Pancreatitis
Mild form	Severe form
Minimal pancreatic/systemic dysfunction	Systemic and pancreatic failure with complications
Pancreatic edema and mild cellular infiltrates Few scattered foci of necrosis in the peripancreatic fat	Extensive fat necrosis, hemorrhage, liquefaction of pancreatic parenchyma and adjacent peripancreatic areas and fascial planes
Relatively homogeneous enhancement with mild peripancreatic fat stranding/fluid	Non-enhancing necrotic areas (</> 30%) within the pancreatic parenchyma
	Ill-defined peripancreatic collections obliterate the adjacent fat and dissect the fascial planes, such as Gerota's fascia, resulting in the collections in the pararenal space anteriorly, in bilateral flanks, and the pelvis and groin regions via psoas
< 4 weeks—Acute peripancreatic fluid collection Homogeneous density, no wall, conforms to the fascial planes	*< 4 weeks—Acute necrotic collection* Multiloculated intra/extrapancreatic necrotic collections without any discernable wall
> 4 weeks—Pseudocyst Well-defined, homogeneously fluid density, round to oval collection, usually due to pancreatic duct disruption	*> 4 weeks—Walled-off Necrosis (WON)* Walled-off heterogeneously enhancing intra/extrapancreatic necrotic collections (Figure 1.33b)

Intermediate forms of pancreatitis may occur depending on the imaging findings and presentation (Figure 1.33b).

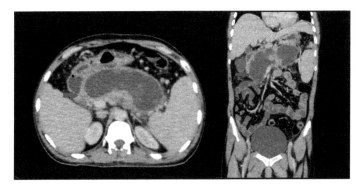

Figure 1.33b CECT abdomen depicts reduced pancreatic parenchyma, replaced by a large, well-defined walled-off peripherally enhancing multiloculated, hypoattenuating collection showing few enhancing septations within, seen in the peripancreatic region with significant adjacent fat stranding and extending locally walled off necrosis.

Complications

- *Emphysematous Pancreatitis*: secondary infection with gas-forming organisms.

- Vascular complications such as pseudoaneurysms, portal, and splenic vein thrombosis.

Differentiating pancreatitis depending on its severity (Tables 1.21 and 1.22).

Table 1.21: **Severity of Pancreatitis**

Mild Acute Pancreatitis	Moderate Acute Pancreatitis	Severe Acute Pancreatitis
No organ failure No local/systemic complications	Transient single/multiple organ failure or local/systemic complications	Persistent single/multiple organ failure or local/systemic complications
No testing and imaging required	May resolve without intervention	Intervention required
Discharged during the early phase. Mortality rare	Mortality depends on the involvement, not severe	High mortality rate

Table 1.22: **Imaging Findings on Various Modalities**

USG   Focal/diffusely enlarged hypoechoic pancreas. Pancreatic echogenicity varies with

- Time of study-reduced echogenicity after 2–5 days of symptom onset
- Amount of peripancreatic fat, increases with age along with its echogenicity
- Degree of extrapancreatic spread
- Hemorrhage
- Calcifications due to chronic pancreatitis

CT   Initial CT should be done 3–4 days after the onset of symptoms
To evaluate the extent of the disease to assess the severity
To identify the etiology
For guided therapeutic interventions

MRI   Enlarged homogeneous gland is low signal on T1WI and high on T2WI. Dilated PD is hyperintense on T2WI
Enlarged heterogeneous pancreas with shaggy and irregular contour
Peripancreatic high signal on T1WI fat suppressed sequences due to fat necrosis and hemorrhage

Findings

- Patchy areas of absent enhancement due to liquefactive necrosis.

- Ill-defined peripancreatic collections obliterate the adjacent fat and dissect the fascial planes, such as Gerota's fascia, resulting in the collections in the pararenal space anteriorly, in bilateral flanks, and the pelvis and groin regions via psoas.

Modified CT Severity Index (Table 1.23)

Table 1.23: **Grading of Pancreatitis**

Points	Pancreatic Inflammation	Necrosis
0	Normal	Nil
2	Pancreatic parenchymal abnormalities	< 30%
4	Pancreatic and peripancreatic abnormalities	> 30%

Additional two points for complexities such as vascular complications and fluid collections in pleural and peritoneal cavities, etc.

The score is graded as mild (0–2), severe (8–10), and moderate, if in between.

Case 26   Chronic Pancreatitis

Case: A 65-year-old alcoholic male with vague abdominal pain (Figure 1.34).

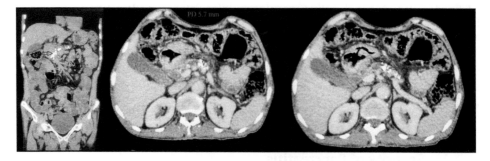

Figure 1.34   CECT abdomen depicts calcifications in atrophied pancreas with mild duct dilatation.

Discussion

Chronic pancreatitis can be described as a persistent and progressive inflammatory disease of the pancreas with irreversible structural changes resulting in pain as well as exocrine and endo-crine abnormalities. The most common causes include alcoholism, gallstones, drug-induced, idiopathic, and hereditary pancreatitis. It may be focal or diffuse and usually presents with pain, vomiting, unintentional weight loss, malabsorption, and development of diabetes mellitus. The normal pancreas is echogenic compared to the liver, and its fatty replacement increases with age. The retroperitoneal location of the pancreas, overlying bowel gas, and operator-dependent nature render the sonography of the pancreas difficult. On CT scan, the normal pancreas appears homogeneous and smoothly lobulated.

Imaging reveals ductal dilatation, calcifications, strictures, pancreatic texture, and involvement of adjacent regions. Sonography depicts a heterogeneous pancreas in the early stages followed by irregularly dilated PD with calcific foci and an atrophied pancreas in the late stages. Complications such as pseudocysts and obstructive lesions can be delineated better on CT/MRCP. NCCT abdomen can detect calcifications. CECT outlines vascular complications, pseudocysts, and focal lesions along with ductal evaluation for planning surgical interventions.

Fat-suppressed T1WI shows a loss of signal intensity. MRCP shows the calcific foci as filling defects and the beaded appearance of a pancreatic duct due to alternate strictures and dilatation.

Differential Diagnosis

- Carcinoma pancreas
- Intraductal papillary mucinous neoplasm (IPMN)
- Autoimmune pancreatitis
- Groove/Paraduodenal pancreatitis

Management

- Conservative management for pain (analgesics)
- Nutritional support and enzyme replacement
- Diabetes control
- Surgical interventions for complications

Case 27 Pancreas Divisum

A 22-year-old male with recurrent pancreatitis (Figure 1.35).

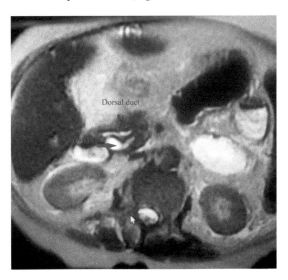

Figure 1.35 MRI abdomen depicts the dorsal pancreatic duct crossing anterior to the common bile duct (CBD) and emptying separately into the minor papilla.

Discussion

Pancreas divisum/divided pancreas, with failure of fusion of ventral and dorsal pancreatic buds and their respective ducts, is a frequent congenital variant of the pancreatic ductal anatomy (Figure 1.35). The dorsal duct drains most of the pancreatic parenchyma through the minor papilla and predisposes to pancreatitis due to inefficient drainage of secretions. The ventral duct joins CBD, drains a portion of the pancreatic head, and uncinate process through the major papilla.

Management
Acute recurrent pancreatitis may require sphincterotomy, balloon dilatation, or stent placement in the duct.

Case 28 Mediastinal Extension of Pseudopancreatic Cyst
A 30-year-old male with abdominal discomfort, dyspnea, and elevated amylase (Figure 1.36).

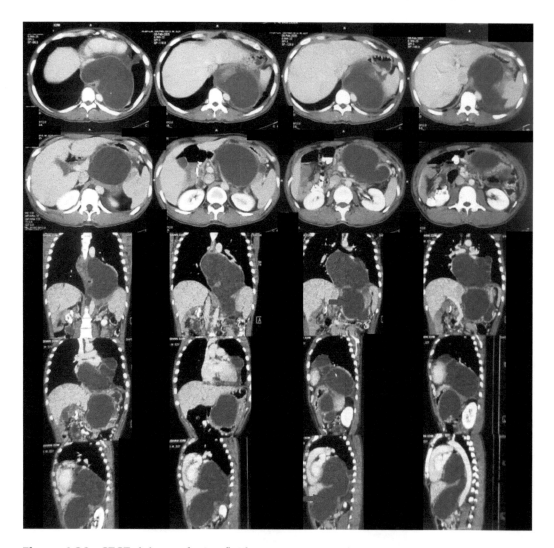

Figure 1.36   CECT abdomen depicts fluid containing a pseudopancreatic cyst (arrow) extending to the chest (star).

Discussion
Pseudocyst is a thin-walled fluid collection lined by granulation or fibrous tissue around the pancreas as a sequelae of trauma, acute or chronic pancreatitis. Extension of pancreatic pseudocyst (PP) into mediastinum may result in compression symptoms such as chest pain, dyspnea, and dysphagia. The fluid collection traverses the path of least resistance and extends to the posterior mediastinum (through esophageal or aortic hiatus) or anterior/middle mediastinum (through foramen of Morgagni/IVC hiatus).

Chest X-ray shows lower mediastinal widening, retro/para cardiac opacity, and pleural effusion.

CECT depicts thin-walled peripherally enhancing hypodense fluid collection extending ectopically into the mediastinum. MRI/MRCP shows TI hypointense and T2 hyperintense lesions and better delineates the direct communication between MPD and mediastinal pseudocyst, confirming the pancreatic origin of the lesion.

Differential Diagnosis

Cystic lesions of the pancreas and mediastinal cystic lesions.

Management

- Conservative

- Image-guided/endoscopic internal/external drainage in symptomatic patients with complications.

Case 29 Pancreatic Lipomatosis

A 34-year-old female with vague abdominal discomfort (Figure 1.37).

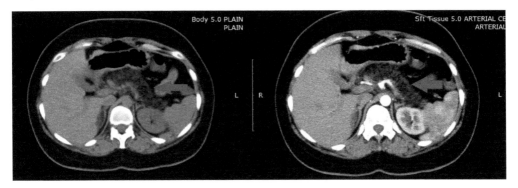

Figure 1.37 NCCT and CECT abdomen depicts an enlarged pancreas replaced with low-density fat tissue with normal pancreaticobiliary ductal system.

Discussion

It is a benign entity frequently a/w obesity and aging. Sonography reveals a hyperechoic pancreas that is difficult to discern from the adjacent tissues. NCCT depicts a diffusely enlarged hypodense fatty pancreas, with the acinar tissue and ductal structures strands replacing the pancreas, compressing the duodenum, and displacing the small bowel anteriorly. CECT reveals heterogeneous enhancement of the remaining pancreatic parenchyma. MRI shows high signal intensity on TI- and T2WI and may show loss of signal intensity on opposed-phase T1WI.

Differential Diagnosis

- Lipomatous pseudohypertrophy

- Congenital syndromes such as cystic fibrosis, Shwachman–Diamond syndrome

- Focal lipomatosis simulates neoplastic lesion

- Pancreatic agenesis (disrupted ductal system)

Case 30 Groove Pancreatitis

A 51-year-old alcoholic male presented with abdominal pain and vomiting with elevated amylase and lipase levels (Figure 1.38).

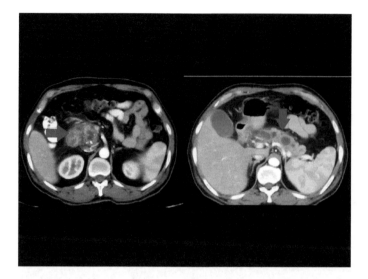

Figure 1.38 CECT abdomen depicts expansion of pancreaticoduodenal groove with loss of fat plane with the mildly bulky pancreatic head by a heterogeneously enhancing sheet-like soft tissue density lesion prominent pancreatic duct, duodenal wall thickening, and intramural cysts. Biopsy ruled out tumor.

Discussion

Paraduodenal pancreatitis, initially known as groove pancreatitis, is chronic fibrotic inflammation of the pancreas between the medial wall of the duodenum and the pancreatic head. The patient may present with epigastric pain, vomiting, and weight loss due to duodenal obstruction.

Two forms:

1. Pure form involves mainly PDG

2. Segmental form with epicenter in the PDG and extension into the pancreatic head

MRCP help confirm the findings of expanded PDG with lesions depicting low T1SI, intramural cysts, and medial duodenal wall thickening on T2WI, smoothly tapered stricture of CBD apart from delayed enhancement of fibrotic tissue. Normal peripancreatic vessels without thrombosis or infiltration on CT.

Differential Diagnosis

- Pancreatic adenocarcinoma (homogeneously hypodense tumor, vascular invasion, high uptake at PET-CT, restricted diffusion on DWI, elevated tumor markers—CA 19-9 and carcinoembryonic antigen).

- Duodenal carcinoma.

- Acute edematous pancreatitis (a/w peripancreatic stranding and collection extending into anterior pararenal spaces).

- Duodenitis (Crohn's disease).

- Retroperitoneal sarcoma extending into the groove (anterior displacement of both pancreatic head and duodenum).

Management

Conservative treatment with bed rest, intravenous nutrition, and analgesics.

Whipple's procedure may be required in a few cases.

Case 31 Pancreatic Amyloidosis

A 49-year-old diabetic male patient presented with pain in the abdomen, normal serum amylase, and ketonuria. The patient had a history of left nephrectomy and abnormal RFTs (Figure 1.39).

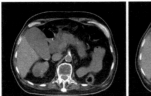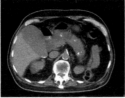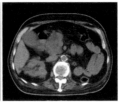

Figure 1.39 NCCT abdomen depicts normal-density, diffusely enlarged pancreas (open arrows) with multiple scattered punctate calcifications, non-dilated pancreatic duct, and CBD. No peripancreatic fat stranding or abnormal fluid accumulation. Left-sided nephrectomy (star) with irregular right renal outline due to multiple cortical cysts in this patient with chronic renal disease.

Discussion

Pancreatic amyloidosis is a rare disease in which abnormal amyloid protein (IAPP-Islet Amyloid Poly Peptide) deposits in the pancreas in patients with type II diabetes mellitus. The risk factors include increasing age, poorly controlled diabetes, and a family history of amyloidosis. It is a cause and also a sequel of type 2 diabetes mellitus. It is usually isolated/focal rather than systemic.

Primary amyloidosis usually lacks a chronic inflammatory process compared to secondary amyloid deposition, resulting from chronic inflammatory or destructive processes in various organs. Sonography depicts a diffusely enlarged hypoechoic pancreas with punctate hyperechogenities representing calcifications. MRI shows a diffusely enlarged pancreas hypointense on both T1- and T2WI. The acute abdomen in this patient was due to diabetic ketoacidosis. Radiologists should be familiar with the appearance of amyloidosis as a high index of suspicion is required for this possibility. Biopsy is confirmative.

Differential Diagnosis

- *Diffuse Pancreatitis*: Presence of pancreatic or peripancreatic fluid collection/fat stranding, pancreatic duct abnormality, clinical history, and enzyme levels.

- *Lymphoma*: Absence of multiple calcifications, presence of lymphadenopathy or other abdominal findings pointing toward lymphoma, biopsy findings.

- *Auto-Immune Pancreatitis*: Hypodense halo or rim sign, smooth pancreatic outline with loss of clefts (sausage-shaped pancreas or featureless pancreatic border), homogeneous enhancement, calcification rare, clinical or imaging findings in the setting of obstructive jaundice, increased IgG4, histology, and response to steroid therapy.

- *Tuberculosis of Pancreas*: Usually inhomogeneously enhancing septated cystic lesion with heterogeneous parenchyma and calcifications involving the mass or the irregularly narrowed pancreatic duct rather than pancreatic parenchyma. Patients usually have lymphadenopathy apart from the involvement of the chest or abdomen. MRI shows hyperintense pancreas and narrowing of the pancreatic duct.

Management

Adequate glycemic control to avert further damage.

Case 32 Pancreatic Transection

A 25-year-old male with h/o trauma and acute epigastric pain (Figure 1.40).

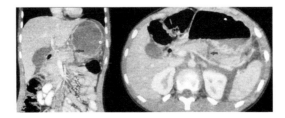

Figure 1.40 CECT abdomen shows linear low attenuation transection line running through pancreatic parenchyma with clear separation of two ends of gland accompanied by free fluid in the abdomen.

Discussion

Pancreas is compressed against the spine in high-force blunt trauma, and seat belt/steering wheel injuries. The pancreas may appear edematous with heterogeneous parenchymal enhancement and depict fluid collections, hematomas, linear branching lacerations, etc. It may be a/w adjacent fat stranding, thickened anterior pararenal fascia, and injuries to other organs, mainly the duodenum. The portal venous phase better assesses the pancreas.

Grading of pancreatic injury (Table 1.24).

Table 1.24: Grading of Pancreatic Injury

Grade	Parenchymal Injury	Duct Disruption
I	Minor contusion, superficial laceration, hematoma	No
II	Major contusion (edematous pancreas)/laceration	No
III	Distal transection (full-thickness tear)	Yes
IV	Proximal transection (also involves ampulla/CBD)	Yes
V	Shattered pancreas	Yes

Management

Surgery

Case 33 Solid Papillary Epithelial Neoplasm

A 20-year-old female with palpable mass and acute epigastric pain (Figure 1.41).

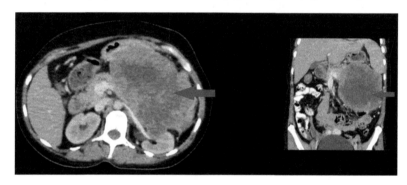

Figure 1.41   CECT abdomen depicts a large, well-circumscribed, heterogeneously enhancing solid-cystic lesion with a few areas of hemorrhage and cystic degeneration in the pancreatic body and tail.

Discussion

Solid papillary epithelial neoplasm (SPEN)/Frantz tumor, an uncommon solid-cystic neoplasm of the pancreas with cystic and hemorrhagic degeneration.

Sonography shows a large, well-circumscribed, heterogeneous mass with echogenic hemor-rhagic areas, papillary projections, and hypoechoic cystic areas. CECT, in addition, reveals a thick enhancing wall with peripheral calcification. MRI depicts T1 and T2 hypointense capsule and hemorrhagic debris showing blooming. The lesion has a propensity to metastasize to the liver, lymph nodes, and omentum but has a favorable prognosis on surgery, mandating early diagnosis.

Differential Diagnosis

This is discussed in Table 1.25.

Table 1.25: Differential Diagnoses of Pancreatic Lesions

	Serous Cystadenoma (SCN)	Mucinous Cystadenoma (MCN)	Solid Papillary Epithelial Neoplasm (SPEN)	Intraductal Papillary Mucinous Neoplasm (IPMN)	Pseudocyst	Cystic Degeneration of Adenocarcinoma	Pancreatic Neuroendocrine Tumors (NETs)
Age	>60 years females	40–60 years females	20–40 years females	50–60 years male	Any	> 60 years males	>50
Location	Head	body/tail	Tail	Head	Anywhere	Head >tail	Body
Associations	Benign	Premalignant	Low-grade malignant potential	High risk of malignancy	Trauma, pancreatitis	Malignancy	Syndromes such as MEN 1, VHL, NF 1
Imaging	Lobulated, microcystic(honeycomb pattern), thin-walled serous fluid, central calcified scar	Macrocystic, unilocular, thick enhancing septae, wall calcification	Well, encapsulated Hemorrhage and cystic degeneration	Multiple unilocular/septated. Main duct type/branched duct type	Fluid density with thin enhancing wall	Hypovascular infiltrative mass with cystic degeneration, vascular invasion, and PD obstruction	Avidly enhancing hypervascular tumors with cystic-necrotic degeneration
Communication between cyst and PD	No	No	No	Yes, MRCP delineates communication	No	No	No

45

Management

Surgery

Case 34 Pancreatic Adenocarcinoma

A 55-year-old male presented with abdominal distension (Figure 1.42).

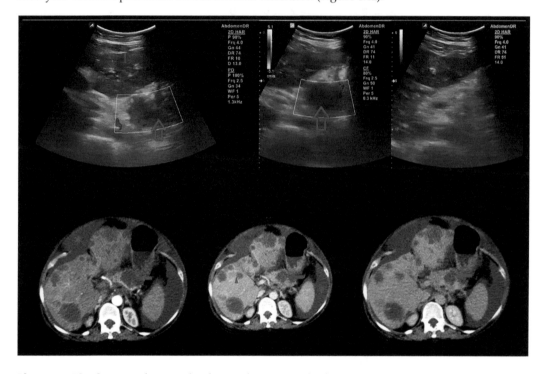

Figure 1.42 Sonography reveals a hypoechoic avascular lesion in the pancreas. CECT abdomen depicts a well-defined heterogeneously hypodense hypovascular lesion (solid arrow) in the distal body and tail of the pancreas. The lesion shows minimal post-contrast enhancement. It also depicts hepatomegaly with subtle surface irregularity and variable-sized hypodense lesions (arrowheads) with post-contrast enhancement in the portal-venous phase. Gross ascites (star) in the pelvic and peritoneal cavity with aortocaval lymph nodal deposit.

Discussion

Pancreatic ductal adenocarcinoma, a deadly malignancy with early metastasis and a high fatality rate, mandates early identification of the extent of the lesion and its spread for efficient patient management.

Patients with pancreatic head tumors may present with double duct sign due to dilated CBD and PD. Endoscopic sonography (EUS) shows an ill-defined, heterogenous hypo/avascular lesion and helps detect and staging the tumors. Due to scirrhous fibrotic content, the lesion is hypointense on T1- and T2WI and enhances less than the normal pancreas. Intense uptake, even in the smallest lesion, is noted on the FDG-PET scan. The malignancy frequently metastasized to the liver and peritoneum.

Differential Diagnosis

This is discussed in Table 1.25.

Management

Palliative therapy and surgery, if no spread.

Case 35 Pancreatic Neuroendocrine Tumors

A 24-year-old male with hypoglycemia and neuroglycopenic symptoms (Figure 1.43).

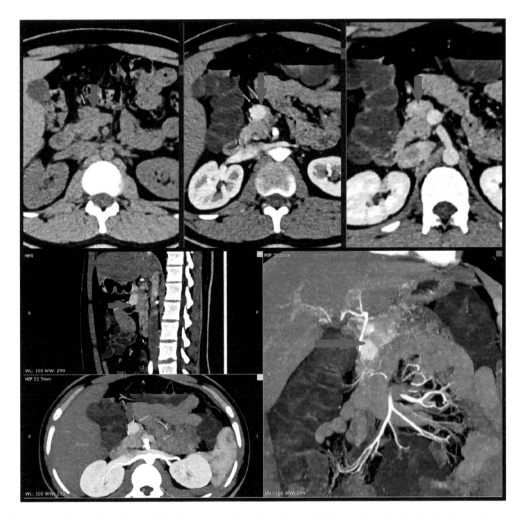

Figure 1.43 CT abdomen depicts intensely enhancing soft tissue density lesion in the anterior surface of the head and uncinate process of the pancreas. The superior pancreaticoduodenal artery, a branch of the common hepatic artery supplies the lesion. Neck sonography revealed two hypervascular lesions in the right parathyroid bed.

Discussion

PaNETs may be functional (release biochemically active substances such as insulin, glucagon, somatostatin, etc.) or non-functional. Insulinoma is the most common, benign, solitary, slow-growing, hypervascular intrapancreatic neuroendocrine islet cell tumor that may have calcifications. The lesion is well-marginated, hypoechoic/dense, and enhances avidly in the arterial phase. The lesion is T1 hypointense, T2 hyperintense, and shows restricted diffusion.

Differential Diagnosis

Hypervascular metastasis (discussed in Table 1.25).

Management

Surgery is curative.

PEDIATRIC SECTION

Case 36 Annular Pancreas

An 11-year-old female presented with abdominal pain and vomiting (Figure 1.44).

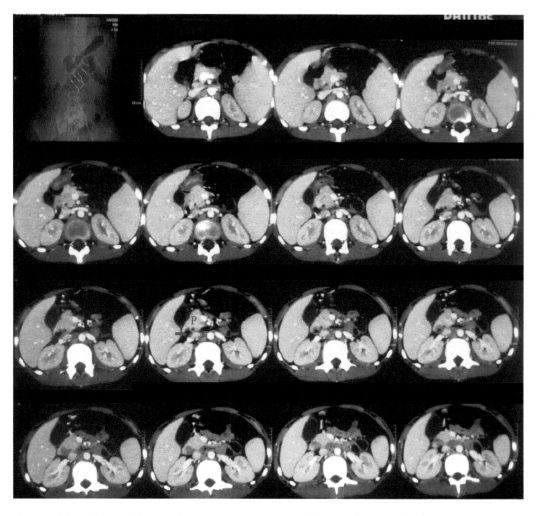

Figure 1.44 CECT abdomen depicts pancreatic tissue (P) encircling the duodenum (arrow) incompletely, giving a crocodile jaw appearance.

Discussion

Annular pancreas is a rare morphological anomaly, with pancreatic tissue encircling the duodenum. It may present in the neonatal period with duodenal obstruction or in adults as asymptomatic or abdominal pain, vomiting, post-prandial fullness, and pancreatitis. It is frequent in males and may be a/w Down's syndrome, Hirschsprung's disease, duodenal atresia, congenital heart disease, etc. A disruption in the pancreatic embryologic development causes failure of the ventral bud to rotate, resulting in developing pancreatic tissue encircling the duodenum in a ring of the pancreas. The encasement can be complete or incomplete (crocodile jaw appearance). The upper GI series shows concentric narrowing along the duodenum's second part with proximal dilatation. CT/MRCP better delineates the pancreatic tissue/ductal abnormality. CBD lies posteromedial to duodenum.

Management

Surgery in symptomatic cases.

Case 37 Hepatoblastoma

A 2-year-old female with abdominal distension and pain (Figure 1.45).

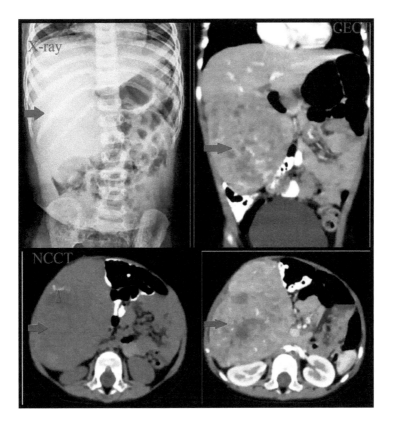

Figure 1.45 X-ray depicts hepatomegaly causing displacement of bowel loops. CT abdomen reveals a large, well-marginated, heterogeneously enhancing lesion with peripheral calcifications and necrotic components, displacing the bowel loops.

Discussion

Hepatoblastoma, the most common primary malignant hepatic neoplasm in the pediatric age group with a slight male predilection, originates from primitive hepatic stem cells and is associated with elevated AFP levels and specific syndromes such as Beckwith Weidmann, Gardner's, familial adenomatosis polyposis, etc.

A large heterogeneously hyperechoic mass is seen on ultrasound. Coarse calcifications are better evaluated with NCCT with heterogeneous enhancement on CECT. T1 and T2WI show heterogeneously enhancing mixed signal intensity lesions owing to significant intratumoral necrosis and hemorrhage. Cross-sectional imaging aids in assessing nodal status, vascular infiltration, and distant metastases with superior resolution on MRI as compared to CT, particularly in cases of vascular invasion, which is seen as a loss of T2 flow-void with intravascular T2 hyperintense thrombus.

The liver is divided into four sections: left lateral (segments 2 and 3), left medial (segments 4a and 4b), right anterior (segments 5 and 8), and right posterior (segments 6 and 7). PRETEXT staging of hepatic tumors depends on the involvement of the number of these four sections. Thorough analysis as per the PRETEXT staging should be done as it inversely correlates with the prognosis. Careful interpretation must be made regarding tumoral thrombus and distant metastases to aid in surgical management.

Differential Diagnosis

■ Hepatic mesenchymal hamartoma

■ Infantile hemangioma

■ Hepatic metastases (from other embryonal tumors—neuroblastoma)

Management

Surgical resection, with pre- and postoperative chemotherapy as required, is the treatment of choice, with liver transplantation being curative in patients without metastases.

Case 38 Choledochal Cyst

A 6-year-old female with acute pancreatitis (Figures 1.46 and 1.47).

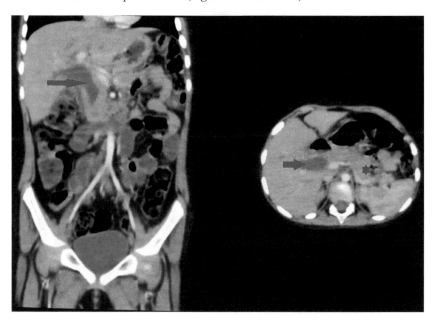

Figure 1.46   CECT abdomen depicts fusiform dilatation of extrahepatic bile ducts (CBD) Type Ic with mildly prominent central IHBR. Bulky body and tail of the pancreas.

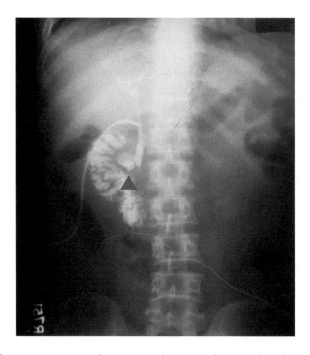

Figure 1.47   Cholangiogram in another patient depicting diverticulum from EHBD—type 2 choledochal cyst.

Discussion

CDCs, congenital cystic dilatation of the biliary tree, usually present with abdominal pain, jaundice, and mass. It is premalignant, may be a/w anomalous pancreaticobiliary junction, and has the propensity to form calculi, cholangitis, rupture (peritonitis), and pancreatitis. Sonography is the initial modality of choice for assessing biliary dilatation. CT scan depicts non-enhancing cystic structure in porta hepatis contiguous with biliary tree. Hepatobiliary scintigraphy evaluates physiological status. ERCP, MRCP, PTC, and intra-operative cholangiography better delineate anatomy.

CDC types (Table 1.26)

Table 1.26: **Types of Choledochal Cysts**

1	Most common: EHBD dilatation (saccular/fusiform)—three types: (a) generalized, (b) localized, and (c) CBD part
2	True diverticulum (saccular outpouching) from supraduodenal EHBD
3	Protruded intramural segment of distal CBD into the duodenum (choledochocele). Similar to santorinocele
4	Fusiform dilatation of EHBD with IHBD extension Multiple dilatations/cysts of EHBD
5	Multiple dilatations of IHBD (Caroli's disease)
6	Cystic duct dilatation

Differential Diagnosis

- Other causes of biliary tree dilatation include biliary stricture, calculi, etc.

- Enteric duplication cysts

- Pancreatic cystic lesions

Management

- Depends on the type and symptoms.

- Surgical resection (Roux-en-Y hepaticojejunostomy)

SUGGESTED READINGS

Chernyak, V., Fowler, K. J., Kamaya, A., et al. Liver imaging reporting and data system (LI-RADS) version 2018: Imaging of hepatocellular carcinoma in at-risk patients. *Radiology* 2018;289:3, 816–830.

Drake, R. L., Vogl, A. W., Mitchell, A. W. M., Tibbitts, R., & Richardson, P. (2020). *Gray's Atlas of Anatomy E-Book*. Elsevier Health Sciences.

Eisenhauer, E. A., Therasse, P., Bogaerts, J., et al. New response evaluation criteria in solid tumours: Revised RECIST guideline (version 1.1). *Eur J Cancer* 2009;45:228–247.

Kozar, R., Crandall, M., Shanmuganathan, K., et al. Organ injury scaling 2018 update: Spleen, liver, and kidney. *J Trauma Acute Care Surg*. 2018;85(6):1119–1122. doi:10.1097/ta.0000000000002058.

Lee, J. K. T. (2006). *Computed Body Tomography with MRI Correlation*. Lippincott Williams & Wilkins.

Moore, E. E., Cogbill, T. H., Malangoni, M. A., Jurkovich, G. J., Shackford, S. R., Champion, H. R., & McAninch, J. W. Organ injury scaling. *Surg Clin North Am*. 1995;75(2):293–303. doi: 10.1016/s0039-6109(16)46589-8.

2 Gastrointestinal Tract

INTRODUCTION

Embryology

The primitive gut develops when a part of the yolk sac is integrated into the embryo due to the embryo's cephalocaudal and lateral folding. The yolk sac and the allantois stay outside the embryo. The primitive gut is a blind-ended tube on the embryo's cephalic end as the foregut, the caudal end as the hindgut, and the middle part as the midgut, which is attached to the yolk sac via the vitelline duct (yolk stalk) (Table 2.1 and Figure 2.1).

Foregut

The tracheoesophageal septum separates with the ventral part forming the respiratory system and the dorsal part forming GIT. The esophagus develops from the foregut. Initially, the length is short but later elongates due to the formation of the neck, the descent of the diaphragm, and the enlargement of pleural cavities. Epithelium and glands are derived from endoderm and musculature

Table 2.1: **Derivatives of Gut**

Foregut	Midgut	Hindgut
Celiac axis	SMA	IMA
Trachea, respiratory tract, pharynx, esophagus, stomach, liver, GB, bile ducts, pancreas, and proximal duodenum	Distal duodenum, jejunum, ileum, cecum, ascending colon, and proximal two-thirds of transverse colon	Distal one-third of the transverse colon, descending colon, sigmoid colon, rectum and urogenital sinus

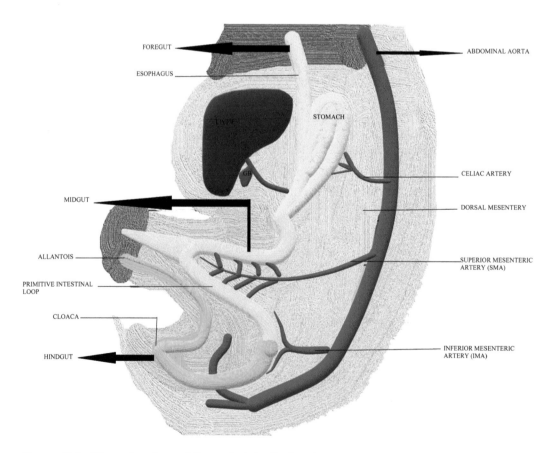

Figure 2.1 The embryology of the gastrointestinal system.

DOI: 10.1201/9781003452034-2

from mesoderm. Mesenchyme surrounding the upper two-thirds of the esophagus forms striated muscle, and mesenchyme surrounding the lower one-third forms smooth muscle. Failure of tracheoesophageal septum results in TEF+/− esophageal atresia.

The stomach forms as a fusiform dilatation of the foregut. The first and second 90° clockwise rotation in longitudinal and transverse axes alters the position of vagus nerves, changes the orientation of their surfaces, and forms lesser and greater sac/omental bursa. The first part and the upper half of the second part of the duodenum are derived from the foregut. Most of the duodenum is retroperitoneal because the mesoduodenum fuses with the peritoneum of the posterior abdominal wall.

Midgut

Between the fifth and tenth weeks of pregnancy, the midgut loop elongates by herniating into the umbilical cord and communicating to the yolk sac by the vitellointestinal duct.

First, the midgut rotates 90° counterclockwise around the superior mesenteric artery. Then, it enters the abdominal cavity again, rotating 180° anticlockwise. The cecum is located in the right upper quadrant of the abdominal cavity after this complex 270° anticlockwise rotation (90° + 180°). The cecum is then pushed down into its final place as the colon expands. Proximal and narrower distal parts of the caecal bud form the caecum and appendix, respectively.

- Omphalocele results from failure of the midgut loop to return to the abdomen.

- Meckel's diverticulum is a persistent remnant of the vitelline duct, forming a blind pouch on the antimesenteric border of the ileum.

- Malrotation occurs if the midgut undergoes only partial rotation.

Hindgut

The dorsal subdivision of the cloaca (primitive rectum) forms the rectum and upper two-thirds of the anal canal. The lower part of the anal canal is derived from the ectoderm and develops from proctodeum. The pectinate line (anal valves) forms the junction of endodermal and ectodermal parts (Table 2.2).

Enteric nervous system constitutes ganglion neuron networks derived from neural crest cells.

1. Myenteric (Auerbach) plexus—Between the inner circular and the outer longitudinal muscle layers.

2. Submucosal (Meissner) plexus—Situated adjacent to the mucosal layer.

    The duodenum, ascending colon, descending colon, and rectum become retroperitoneal after the rotation of the gut is completed by fusion of their mesenteries with the posterior abdominal wall compared to the mesentery of the small intestine mesentery, transverse mesocolon, and pelvic mesocolon which persists as original.

Anatomy

The *esophagus* is a muscular tube that is 24–30 cm long and connects the pharynx to the stomach. It has inner circular and outer longitudinal muscles that contract and relax in coordinated peristaltic waves to push food downward. The esophagus has four natural constrictions along its length—near the upper esophageal sphincter (UES), aortic constriction, left atrium constriction, and diaphragmatic hiatus. It is innervated by the vagus nerve, which controls the involuntary muscular contractions needed for swallowing and peristalsis.

Table 2.2: **Anal Canal Division**

Anal canal	Upper two-thirds of anal canal	Lower one-third of anal canal
Origin	Endoderm of hindgut (primitive rectum)	Ectodermal proctodeum (anal pit)
Arterial supply	Superior rectal artery (SMA)	Inferior rectal artery (Internal pudendal artery, and branch of internal iliac artery)
Venous drainage	Portal vein via superior rectal vein	IVC via inferior rectal vein
Nerve supply	Autonomic	Somatic
Epithelial lining	Columnar	Stratified squamous

The *stomach* is a vital organ in the digestive system, located in the upper left part of the abdominal cavity, between the esophagus and small intestine just below the diaphragm. It comprises the cardia, fundus, body, pylorus, and lower esophageal and pyloric sphincter.

The *small intestine* is a long, coiled tube extending from the stomach to the large intestine in the central and lower abdomen. The small intestine has a highly folded internal surface covered in tiny finger-like projections called villi and even smaller structures called microvilli, which increase the absorptive area of the small intestine. It contains a network of lymphatic vessels called lacteals, which help absorb dietary fats and fat-soluble vitamins. It consists of duodenum, jejunum, and ileum.

Duodenum (25 cm) in length, C-shaped part of the small intestine with the head of the pancreas enclosed in its concavity. It lies opposite to the L1, L2, and L3 vertebrae and is divided into four parts:

1. Superior (first) part, 5 cm long

2. Descending (second) part, 7.5 cm long

3. Horizontal (third) part, 10 cm long

4. Ascending (fourth) part, 2.5 cm long

The fourth part is continuous with the jejunum at duodenojejunal flexure at the level of the L2 vertebra. The interior of the second part of the duodenum presents the major and minor duodenal papillae.

The major duodenal papilla is located 8–10 cm distal to the pylorus, marking the junction of embryonic foregut and midgut. On its summit, the common hepatopancreatic duct opens. The minor duodenal papilla is placed 2 cm proximal to the major duodenal papilla, and its summit marks the accessory pancreatic duct opening. The suspensory ligament of Trietz is a fibromuscular band that suspends the duodenojejunal flexure from the right crus of the diaphragm. It fixes the duodenojejunal flexure and prevents it from being dragged down. It is an important landmark in the radiological diagnosis of incomplete rotation or malrotation of the small intestine.

Jejunum and ileum form the small intestine and extend from the duodenojejunal flexure to the ileocaecal junction. Its upper two-fifths form the jejunum, and the lower three-fifths form the ileum. The jejunum and ileum are suspended from the posterior abdominal wall by mesentery.

Large intestine spans from the ileocaecal junction to the anus. It is about 1.5 m long. It is divided into the caecum, the ascending colon, the right colic flexure, the transverse colon, the left colic flexure, descending colon, the sigmoid colon, the rectum, and the anal canal. Vermiform appendix is a small blind pouch in the angle between the caecum and the terminal part of the ileum.

The longitudinal muscle coat forms only a thin layer in the large intestine. The greater part of it forms three ribbon-like bands called the taeniae coli. Small bags of peritoneum filled with fat, called appendices epiploicae, are scattered over the surface of the large intestine, except for the appendix, the caecum, and the rectum. It comprises a series of pouches/dilatations (sacculations or haustrations) in the wall of the caecum and colon between the teniae.

It is adapted for storage of matter reaching it from the small intestines and for absorption of fluid and solutes. The epithelium is absorptive (columnar), but villi are absent. The presence of numerous solitary lymphatic follicles protects against bacteria present in the lumen of the intestine.

Caecum communicates with the ascending colon superiorly, with the ileum at the ileocaecal orifice, guarded by the ileocaecal valve, and with the appendix posteromedially. The caecum is almost surrounded by the peritoneum in the majority.

The *appendix* is a narrow worm-like diverticulum arising from the caecum's posteromedial wall with an average length of 9 cm and a diameter of 6 mm. All three teniae of the caecum converge to the base of the appendix, guiding the surgeon to search for the appendix during appendicectomy. The body is a narrow tubular part between the base and the tip. The tip is the least vascular distal blind end. Retrocaecal is the most standard position. The appendix is suspended by a small triangular fold of the peritoneum called the mesentery of the appendix or mesoappendix. The appendicular artery runs within its free margin.

Ascending Colon extends from the caecum to the inferior surface of the right lobe of the liver, where it bends to the left to form the hepatic (right colic) flexure. It is nearly 12.5 cm long, located in the right paracolic gutter, and covered by peritoneum on the front and sides, binding it to the posterior abdominal wall.

Transverse Colon extends from the right colic flexure (in the right lumbar region) to the left colic flexure (in the left hypochondriac region) and is usually U-shaped. It is the most mobile part of the large intestine, nearly 50 cm long, suspended from the posterior abdominal wall by the transverse mesocolon.

Descending Colon extends from the left colic flexure and becomes continuous with the sigmoid colon at the level of the pelvic brim. It is nearly 25 cm long, covered by the peritoneum on the front and sides, which fixes it in the left paracolic gutter and iliac fossa.

Sigmoid or Pelvic Colon extends from the lower end of the descending colon at the left pelvic inlet to the pelvic surface of the third piece of sacrum, where it becomes continuous with the rectum. It is about 37.5 cm in length. It is an S-shaped, so-called sigmoid colon. The sigmoid colon is suspended from the pelvic wall by the peritoneal fold called sigmoid mesocolon, which has an inverted V-shaped attachment/root.

Rectum is about 12 cm long distal part of the large intestine (without characteristic taenia coli, sacculations, and appendices epiploicae) that lies between the sigmoid colon and the anal canal. It is located in the posterior part of the lesser pelvis in front of the lower sacrum and the coccyx and behind the urinary bladder in the male and the uterus in the female. The rectum presents two anteroposterior (sacral and perineal) and three lateral curvatures (upper, middle, and lower lateral). It has temporary and four permanent *(Houston's valves)* mucosal folds. The upper one-third of the rectum is covered by the peritoneum on the front and sides, *the* middle one-third is covered by the peritoneum on the front, and the lower one-third of the rectum is not covered by the peritoneum at all.

Anal Canal is the large intestine's terminal part (3.8 cm long), located in the anal triangle of the perineum between the right and left fat-filled ischiorectal fossae. It begins at the *anorectal junction*, passes downward and backward, and opens at the anal orifice. It is surrounded by an involuntary internal anal sphincter (IAS) and a voluntary external anal sphincter (EAS), whose tone keeps the anal canal closed except during the defecation.

The anal canal is divided into upper and lower parts by the pectinate line. The upper part of the anal canal presents the various mucous folds named anal columns (columns of Morgagni) and anal valves (valves of Morgagni), and anal sinuses, which are vertical recesses between the anal columns and above the anal valves. The white line of Hilton demarcates the mucocutaneous junction.

Injury to EAS during surgery (episiotomy)—fecal incontinence (Table 2.3).

Table 2.3: **Vascular Supply of the Gastrointestinal System**

Esophagus	Proximal	Inferior thyroid artery
	Mid/thoracic	Terminal bronchial arteries
	Distal	Left gastric and left phrenic arteries
Stomach	Lesser curvature	Left gastric artery (celiac artery) Right gastric artery (Proper hepatic artery)
	Greater curvature	Right gastroepiploic artery (gastroduodenal artery) Left gastroepiploic artery (Splenic artery)
	Fundus	5–7 short gastric arteries (Splenic artery)
Duodenum	Up to the level of bile duct opening	Superior pancreaticoduodenal artery
	Below the level of bile duct opening	Inferior pancreaticoduodenal artery
Jejunum and ileum		Jejunal and ileal branches of SMA
Caecum and colon		Branches of SMA and IMA
Appendix		Appendicular artery (branch of the inferior division of the ileocolic artery)
Rectum and anus		Superior rectal artery (branch of IMA) Middle rectal arteries (branch of the anterior division of the internal iliac artery) Inferior rectal arteries (branch of the internal pudendal artery) Median sacral artery (branch of the abdominal aorta)

Normal Variant

- Chiladiti's sign

Anomalous interposition of the colonic loop between the diaphragm and the liver that simulates pneumoperitoneum.

PATHOLOGIES

STOMACH

Case 39 Trichobezoar

Trichobezoars (ball of hair) in stomach are common in patients with psychiatric illness (Figure 2.2).

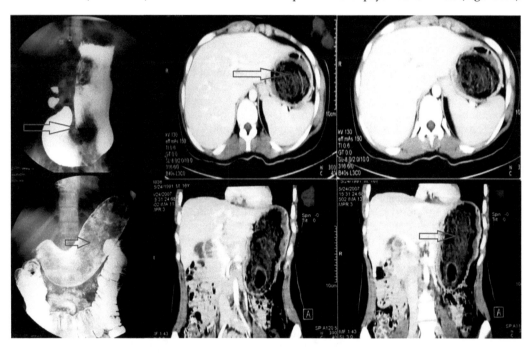

Figure 2.2 Barium studies and CECT depict non-enhancing heterogeneous mass with mottled gas pattern in the stomach.

Discussion

Bezoars are collections of inedible content, such as hairs (trichobezoar), fruits (phytobezoar), etc., that are resistant to digestion and peristalsis, with a propensity to stay in the stomach. A hairball can form over a long period. Extension of a hairball in the small bowel is known as Rapunzel syndrome. They are frequent in adolescent females, especially those with a history of psychiatric ailment, trichotillomania, and trichophagia. The patient presents with anorexia, vomiting, early satiety, bloating, weight loss, and alopecia. Complications include mechanical small bowel obstruction (SBO), obstructive jaundice, perforation, and peritonitis.

A plain X-ray reveals a distended stomach with a mottled gas pattern. Barium studies show an intraluminal filling defect; barium fills the crevices with the mottled gas pattern. An echogenic mass with posterior acoustic shadowing, with absent peristalsis, is noted on sonography. CT accurately delineates the dimensions of the non-enhancing heterogeneous lesion with entrapped air and food debris. Ascites and free air may be seen in cases of perforation.

Management

- Endoscopic removal

- Surgery

Case 40 Gastric Outlet Obstruction due to Duodenal Thickening

A 56-year-old male with vomiting and abdominal fullness (Figure 2.3).

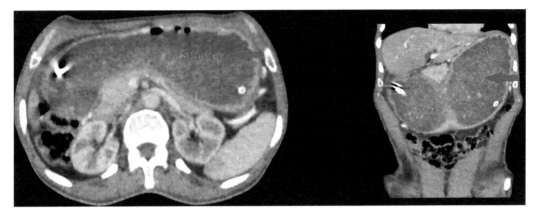

Figure 2.3 CECT abdomen depicts irregular asymmetrically enhancing duodenal thickening due to malignancy causing duodenal narrowing with a massively distended stomach causing GOO.

Discussion

Massive dilatation of the stomach may be seen depending on the degree of gastric outlet obstruction due to various benign and malignant etiologies, including infections, inflammatory diseases, neoplasms, etc. Patients often present with symptoms of nausea, vomiting, fullness, and weight loss.

Plain X-ray shows a nonspecifically distended stomach pushing down the colon without air in the duodenum. Upper GI endoscopy is better for peptic ulcer disease. CT is the preferred method of investigation to evaluate the cause of GOO. High degrees of obstruction are associated with an increased risk of ischemia or perforation. Various etiologies for GOO include:

- Pyloric stenosis and webs—Narrowing without thickened folds
- *Gastritis*: Thickened gastric folds
- *Pancreatitis*: Extent with scoring is easily delineated.
- *Volvulus*: Differentiates between organoaxial and mesenteric axial types.
- *Carcinoma/Lymphoma*: Enhancement of exophytic mass/thickening
- Post-op gastric strictures and scarring after bariatric surgery

Differential Diagnosis

Gastroparesis may show similar gastric dilatation; however, a lesion at the transition zone favors GOO, while gastric wall pneumatosis may be seen in gastroparesis.

Management

Depending on the cause of the disease, passage of the nasogastric tube may resolve gastroparesis, while proper treatment is needed for GOO due to the abovementioned reasons.

Case 41 Gastric Volvulus

A 77-year-old male presented with sudden abdominal distention and vomiting (Figure 2.4).

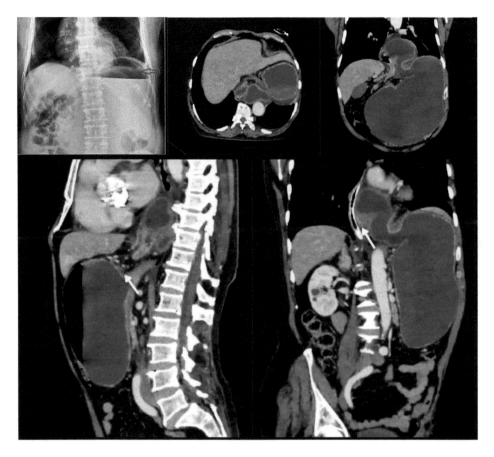

Figure 2.4 Plain X-ray reveals retrocardiac air-fluid level and distended stomach. CECT scan abdomen revealed the abnormal position of the gastroesophageal and gastroduodenal junction at the same level with the inability to pass the nasogastric tube—mesenteric axial gastric volvulus with para-esophageal hiatus hernia.

Discussion

Gastric volvulus is at least 180° twisting of the stomach on its mesentery owing to abnormally long mesentery or abnormal suspensory ligaments, resulting in bowel obstruction. The patient presents with symptoms of severe epigastric pain, intractable retching, and inability to pass the nasogastric tube, commonly referred to as the classic triad of Borchardt. It is commonly a/w hiatal hernia.

It can be classified based on

- Degree of rotation </> 180° (partial vs. complete)
- Time of onset (acute vs. chronic)
- Axis of rotation (along the long axis vs. short axis)

Table 2.4 discusses the differences between the two types of volvulus.

Table 2.4: **Types of Volvulus**

Organo-Axial	Mesenterico-Axial
Adults; a/w trauma or para-esophageal hernia	Children
Along the long axis (cardio pyloric line)	Along the short axis (from lesser to greater curvature)
Common, a/w diaphragmatic defects	Rare
Ischemia rare	Ischemia and strangulation common
GC lies superiorly, LC inferiorly	GE junction to right and pylorus to left

CT findings include elevated stomach and abnormal axis of rotation. The third type is mixed.

Differential Diagnosis

■ Hiatal hernia (herniation of part of the stomach into the thorax)

■ Epiphrenic diverticulum

■ Superior displacement of the stomach due to large abdominal mass

■ Postoperative stomach/esophagectomy with gastric pull-through

Management

Surgical repair (stomach detorsion and gastropexy)

Case 42 Gastrointestinal Stromal Tumors

A 39-year-old male with abdominal distension and palpable abdominal mass (Figure 2.5).

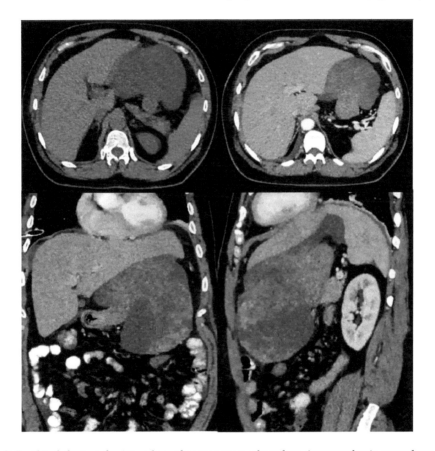

Figure 2.5   CT abdomen depicts a large heterogeneously enhancing exophytic mass from the body of the stomach along the greater curvature. No bowel obstruction was noted.

Discussion

Gastrointestinal Stromal tumors (GISTs) are mesenchymal-origin tumors that can arise anywhere in the GI system, the stomach being the most common location. They usually show a muscular or neural differentiation and can remain relatively asymptomatic until large enough to ulcerate, causing GI bleeds or distant metastasis to the liver and peritoneum. The aggressiveness of GIST directly corresponds to size, with larger tumors having more malignant potential. Patients present with nonspecific GI symptoms such as pain, nausea, and vomiting with GI bleeds in larger-sized tumors. GIST has a familial propensity and is associated with the Carney triad.

CT is most commonly used to detect smaller-sized GISTs and identify calcification or necrosis within the mass. Most GISTs are submucosal exophytic masses and show heterogeneous enhancement. Intramural components may be present, especially in larger tumors. Necrotic areas with ulceration may be filled with air or contrast. Metastases to mesentery and peritoneum, hepatic metastasis, and rarely lung metastasis may be seen. On Barium studies, smaller lesions may be missed; large tumors are often seen as submucosal filling defects with margins forming obtuse angles and preserved mucosal folds. In cases of ulceration within the tumor, contrast extravasation may be seen. MRI shows T1 hypointense and T2 hyperintense mass with enhancement on post-contrast scans. GISTs are PET-avid, and diagnosis is made on immunohistochemistry as these tumors stain positive for KIT (CD 117 and CD 34).

Differential Diagnosis

- Adenocarcinomas (concentric thickening with a bowel obstruction may also have a similar presentation as GIST; however, GIST is rarer in occurrence and usually only involves submucosa).

- True leiomyomas or schwannomas are rare lesions but may present in the GI system.

- Lymphoma (a/w lymphadenopathy, aneurysmal dilatation of bowel with extensive intramural thickening).

Management

GIST has a high recurrence, especially with peritoneal and omental deposits.

Surgical excision is usually done if non-metastatic disease is present. Molecular targeted therapy with Imatinib and Sunitinib has a reasonable success rate.

Case 43 Hiatal Hernia

A 43-year-old patient with postprandial abdominal fullness (Figure 2.6).

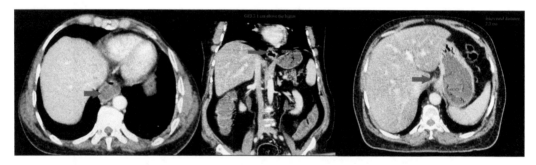

Figure 2.6 CECT abdomen depicts upward migration of GEJ (3.1 cm above the esophageal hiatus), increased intercrural distance (23 mm), and widened angle of His.

Discussion

Hiatal hernia refers to the herniation of the stomach through the esophageal hiatus of the diaphragm. It may be asymptomatic or present with reflux disease, epigastric pain, or abdominal fullness after meals. It may be sliding type (GEJ also herniates with the stomach) or rolling/para-esophageal type (part of the stomach herniates with GEJ in normal location). A plain X-ray may show retrocardiac mass with air-fluid levels. Fluoroscopic studies reveal that the GEJ and > three gastric folds lie above the hiatus. CT depicts a widened esophageal hiatus (normal size is 1.5 cm) with increased distance between the crura and the esophageal wall. The normal 'angle of His' is an acute angle between the abdominal esophagus and the stomach fundus at the GEJ. It widens in a hiatal hernia.

Differential Diagnosis

- Epiphrenic diverticulum
- Retrocardiac lung abscess
- Esophagectomy with gastric pull-up procedure
- Traumatic diaphragmatic rupture

Management

Conservative, if asymptomatic.

  Surgery for symptomatic hernias.

Case 44 Carcinoma Gastroesophageal Junction

A 65-year-old male presented with anorexia, weight loss, dysphagia, abdominal discomfort, and altered LFTs (Figure 2.7).

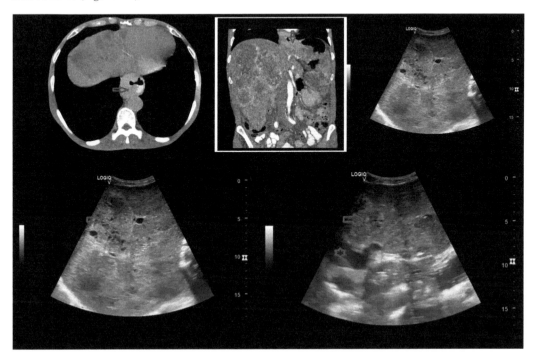

Figure 2.7   Sonography depicted hepatomegaly with multiple heterogeneous lesions (open arrow) involving the entire liver and ascites (star). CECT abdomen shows marked circumferential irregular mural thickening of the GE junction (solid arrow), hepatomegaly with heterogeneously enhancing lesions (open arrow) involving almost the entire liver, and infiltrating adjacent structures with lymphadenopathy.

Discussion

GE junction tumor, mainly adenocarcinoma, occurs distally, where the lower esophagus's squamous epithelial cells migrate to the gastric fundus's columnar epithelial cells. The risk factors include reflux esophagitis, Barrett's esophagitis, smoking, obesity, etc. The patient may present with dysphagia (initially to solids and progressing to liquids), anorexia, and weight loss. The tumor is usually diagnosed at later stages after dissemination of cancer to the liver and lymph nodes.

  Sonography and CT help delineate the extent of the lesion, which is further confirmed by endoscopic biopsy. Peri-esophageal invasion can be seen by evaluating the loss of adjacent fat planes and arc of contact with the aorta (> 90° signifying invasion). Endosonography can be done to stage the tumor as all five layers of the esophagus are well visualized. For all types of esophageal tumors, staging is done based on TNM classification, and localization is done based on the distance of the tumor epicenter from incisors. It is classified as cervical esophageal cancer, upper, mid, or lower (tumors up to 2 cm in the gastric cardia) thoracic esophageal cancer.

Management

- Chemotherapy is usually unsatisfactory. Liver and GE junction resection surgery may be done in a few cases. Interventional radiology is the mainstay treatment if the patient has multiple liver lesions.

- Transarterial chemoembolization (TACE) is used, though only transarterial infusion is preferred as embolization may result in stomach perforation.

- Arterial microsphere embolization is safe and provides better results with reduced tumor size. Embosphere made of acrylic acid and gel polymerization is a permanent agent with reduced toxicity.

SMALL BOWEL

Case 45 Hollow Viscous Perforation

A 39-year-old patient presented with a rigid, acute abdomen (Figure 2.8).

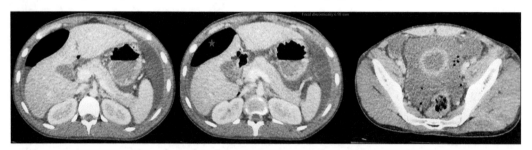

Figure 2.8 CECT abdomen reveals moderate to gross ascites (open arrow) with multiple coarse air locules/foci in perihepatic (star), paracolic, peritoneal, and pelvic cavities, along with mesentery and omental fat stranding. Focal discontinuity in the anterior wall of the first part of the duodenum, extending up to an air locule (solid arrow).

Discussion

Peptic ulcer perforation is the most common cause of hollow viscous perforation (gastric and duodenum). Other causes include trauma, iatrogenic, Helicobacter Pylori infections, steroids, NSAIDs, and necrotic malignancy. The duodenum is prone to injury due to its retroperitoneal location, firm attachment, and juxtaposition to the spine. Irritation by gastrointestinal contents results in clinical signs of rigidity, guarding, and rebound tenderness. Air collects at the midline, lesser sac, spleen, anterior pararenal space, falciform ligament, and ligamentum teres.

CT helps delineate the location of free air/fluid, discontinuity of bowel wall, mural thickening, and adjacent mesenteric/fat stranding. It also differentiates from the duodenal hematoma, which presents with wall thickening and adjoining fluid (discussed in Chapter 7).

Management

Exploratory Laparotomy

Case 46 Intusussception

A 35-year-old female presented with severe crampy abdominal pain and bloody diarrhea (Figure 2.9).

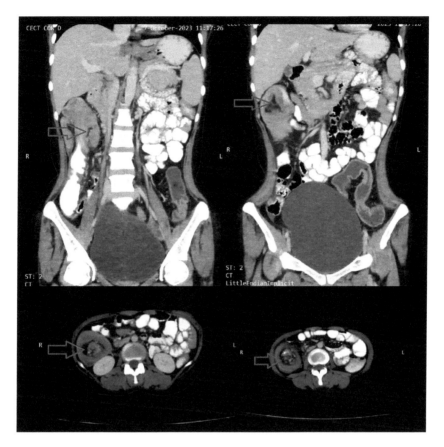

Figure 2.9 CECT abdomen reveals ileal invagination into the colon with lymph nodes in the fat planes of the intussusceptum.

Discussion

Intussusceptum, the proximal bowel loop that invaginates into intussuscipiens, the recipient's distal bowel loop, may result in edema, ischemic changes, obstruction, and necrosis. It is frequent in children, who usually present with acute abdominal pain, vomiting, palpable mass, and hematochezia. It is related to hypertrophied lymphoid tissue; a lead point is not identifiable. It is rare in adults and associated with a lead point, such as benign/malignant tumors, polyps, Meckel's diverticulum, or lymph nodes, as the underlying pathology.

X-ray abdomen depicted a paucity of bowel gas in the right hemiabdomen with features of bowel obstruction (air-fluid levels and proximal bowel dilatation). Fluoroscopy reveals an abnormal bowel loop, giving a pseudokidney appearance. Sonography shows target sign, free fluid, absent vascularity in the intussusceptum, and, if present, a lead point. CT confirms the presence of a lead point, if any. The inner bowel loop and the folded edge of the outer bowel form two concentric enhancing hyperdense rings at the proximal end of intussusception. With distal progression, the compressed central lumen is encircled by the two layers of the outer bowel wall, and the mesentery, or fat and vessels, form a crescent of tissue.

Management

Air enema/water enema

Surgery (laparotomy)

Case 47 Right Paraduodenal Hernia

A 48-year-old male with abdominal pain (Figure 2.10).

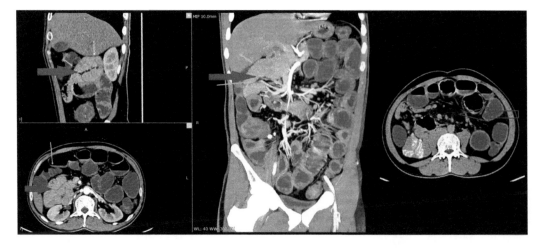

Figure 2.10 CECT abdomen depicts a cluster of small bowel loops (solid arrow) to the right and behind the superior mesenteric vessels and a stretched mesenteric vascular pedicle.

Discussion

Paraduodenal hernia (PDH)—infrequent, congenital aberrations due to defective midgut rotation and failure of mesenteric fusion with the parietal peritoneum. It may present with chronic intermittent abdominal pain that gets relieved with alteration in position and postprandial pain. Herniated bowel loops are usually encapsulated. Bowel obstruction, ischemia, and perforation are frequent with a high mortality.

Types of PDHs (Table 2.5)

Table 2.5: **Types of Paraduodenal Hernias**

Left PDH	Right PDH
Common	Rare (Arrest of the second stage of mid-intestinal rotation)
Fossa of Landzert (defect in the fourth part of duodenum)	Fossa of Waldeyer (defect in the first part of jejunal mesentery)
Midgut lies behind and to the left of SMA and then behind the mesentery of the descending colon	DJ junction is on the right of SMA, SMV is to the left, and the anterior position is to SMA Loops of jejunal vessels move to the right side behind SMA (normally lie on the left side of SMA)
Hernial sac lies posterior to IMV and ascending branch of left colic artery	Hernial sac lies behind SMA, SMV, and the right colic vein
Bowel herniates into the left part of transverse mesocolon within the mesenteric sac (failure of fusion of descending mesocolon to the peritoneum in LUQ)	Bowel herniated into ascending mesocolon (failure of fusion of ascending mesocolon with peritoneum in RLQ)
Situated to the left of the fourth part of the duodenum/anterior pararenal space	Situated below the third part of the duodenum Hernial sac compresses IVC and right psoas muscle Right ureter displaced laterally

NCCT shows hypodense edematous bowel wall due to venous congestion in case of strangulated hernia. Hyperdense bowel wall indicates hemorrhage. Bowel wall and mesenteric hyperemia on CECT help in evaluating bowel wall viability. The whirlpool sign refers to bowel rotation around the mesentery.

Types of internal hernias (Table 2.6)

Table 2.6: **Types of Internal Hernias**

Paraduodenal	Most common; Left and right type Small bowel loops herniating through the congenital mesenteric foramen
Pericecal	Behind (posterolaterally) the cecum and ascending colon Ileal loops protruding through a defect in the cecal mesentery and extending into the right paracolic gutters (d/d appendicitis) Displaces the cecum anteromedially Ileocolic, retrocecal, ileocecal, and paracecal
Foramen of Winslow Predisposition is due to the long mesentery and excessively mobile loops Pain relief with forward bending	Communication between greater and lesser peritoneal cavities, situated beneath the lesser omentum, hepatoduodenal ligament, and portocaval space (portal vein anteriorly and IVC posteriorly) A circumscribed collection of gas-filled loops situated anterolateral and stretching of mesenteric vessels through the foramen (d/d cecal volvulus)
Sigmoid-related hernias	Sacculated ileal loops in LLQ and displacement of sigmoid colon to the right. Maybe a/w mesenteric vessel congestion, fat stranding, and strangulation Types—Intersigmoid, trans-mesosigmoid, intra-mesosigmoid
Transmesenteric	Common in children and are iatrogenic/post-surgery in adults Types—trans-mesocolic, trans-mesenteric, and Peterson Clustered bowel loops in the periphery of the peritoneal cavity with posteroinferior displacement of the transverse colon Lack of omental fat between bowel loops and anterior abdominal wall SMA is displaced to the right with stretching, engorgement, and crowding of mesenteric vessels (d/d small bowel volvulus)
Retroanastomotic	Herniation of bowel loops through a defect related to surgical anastomosis usually occurs during the first postoperative month

Pitfalls

- Clinical suspicion is mandatory as internal hernias are rare as a cause of intestinal obstruction.

- Occasionally, entrapped bowel loops are misdiagnosed as a malignancy, leading to a biopsy and potentially fatal consequences. Hence, it is imperative to CECT with oral contrast, especially in patients without suspicion of intestinal obstruction.

Differential Diagnosis

- Intestinal volvulus
- Adhesions
- Malignancy

Management

Surgery

Case 48 Periampullary Duodenal Diverticula

A 48-year-old female presented with obstructive jaundice (Figure 2.11).

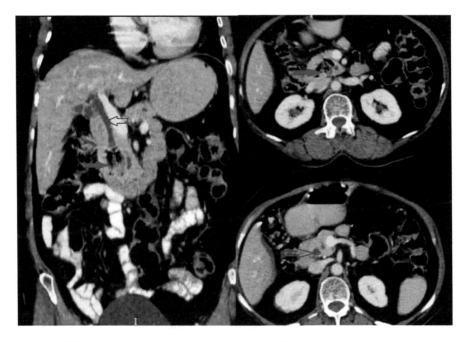

Figure 2.11 CECT abdomen reveals periampullary air-filled duodenal diverticulum arising from the medial wall of the second part of duodenum a/w wall thickening and CBD compression, causing its proximal dilatation.

Discussion

Periampullary duodenal diverticula, an intestinal wall outpouching, is commonly asymptomatic or may present with recurrent hepatobiliary stones, obstructive jaundice, acute pancreatitis, and cholangitis. It may be filled with air, fluid, and enteroliths. It may cause fibrotic inflammation of the papilla or sphincter of Oddi dysfunction or direct CBD compression, resulting in its proximal dilatation. On imaging, it appears as a thin-walled cavitary lesion arising from the medial wall of the second part of the duodenum. Barium studies and MRCP can delineate the contrast-filled outpouching and differentiate it from other pathologies described below. Side-viewing endoscope during ERCP is the gold standard.

Differential Diagnosis

- Pancreatic abscess
- Cystic pancreatic neoplasm
- Necrotic lymphadenopathy
- Todani type II choledochal cyst

Management

Antibiotic course with follow-up evaluation.
   Surgery in cases with complications.

LARGE BOWEL

Case 49 Sigmoid Volvulus

A 70-year-old male with abdominal distention and not passing flatus (Figure 2.12).

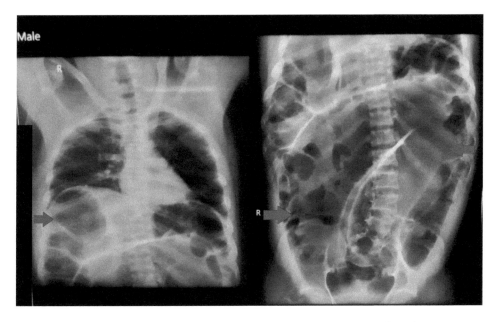

Figure 2.12   Plain X-ray depicts an inverted U-shaped distended loop without haustrations.

Discussion

Sigmoid volvulus is an aberrant twisting of the sigmoid colon along its fixed mesentery resulting in closed-loop obstruction, the risk factors being the long mesentery, chronic constipation, psychiatric illness, and previous abdominal surgery. Plain X-ray shows an inverted U-shaped distended loop without haustrations, elevated hemidiaphragm, and the vertical dense white line due to apposed inner walls of the sigmoid colon. Contrast studies show a beak sign due to smooth tapered narrowing at the rectosigmoid junction. CT, in addition, reveals the whirling of mesenteric vessels.

Differential Diagnosis

Table 2.7 differentiates between sigmoid and cecal volvulus.

Table 2.7: **Differentiation between Sigmoid and Cecal Volvulus**

Sigmoid Volvulus	Cecal Volvulus
LLQ/pelvic origin and points toward RUQ	RLQ origin and points toward LUQ
Haustra absent	Haustra present
Dilated colon	Distended small bowel and collapsed distal bowel

Other differentials include

- Acute ileus without any transition point and obstruction due to postoperative status or ischemia (aperistalsis and air-fluid levels seen).

- Ogilvie's colonic pseudo-obstruction and dilated ahaustral colon without any organic etiology.

- Toxic megacolon as a complication of ulcerative colitis with dilated ahaustral transverse colon.

Management

Surgery

Case 50 Colonic Diverticulosis

A 45-year-old obese male with constipation (Figure 2.13).

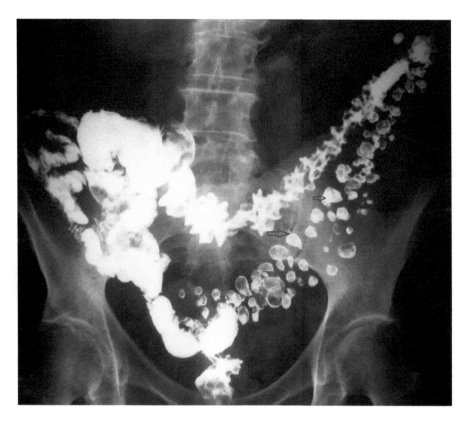

Figure 2.13 Barium study (late film) showing multiple colonic outpouchings and retained barium (arrows).

Discussion

Colonic diverticulosis refers to multiple false diverticula with mesenteric side mucosal herniation due to high intraluminal pressure, chronic constipation, and straining. Myochosis coli refers to a shortened and hypertrophied colon. It is common in the obese population, and the incidence increases with age, the most common site being the sigmoid colon, followed by the descending colon. Patients may be asymptomatic or present with constipation and left-sided abdominal pain. It may get complicated as diverticulitis, the diverticular inflammation with adjacent fat stranding, air locules, and extraluminal fluid. Barium-filled outpouchings are noted in fluoroscopic studies. CT shows outpouchings lined by gas, and virtual colonography shows complete rings of the diverticular neck.

Differential Diagnosis

Polyps—incomplete rings on virtual colonography and contrast outlines the pedicle.

Management

Recommend high-fiber diet.

Case 51 Colo-Colonic Intussusception Caused by Colonic Lipoma

A 50-year-old lady complained of pain in her abdomen (Figure 2.14).

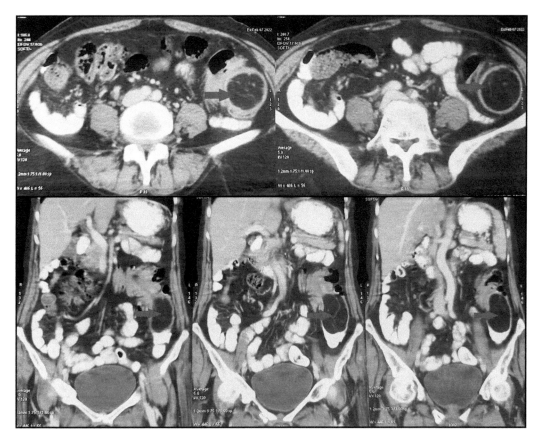

Figure 2.14 CECT abdomen depicts fat density lipoma in the descending colon lumen, acting as a lead point for the intussusception.

Discussion

Colonic lipomas are rare benign mesenchymal submucosal tumors. Small lesions are usually asymptomatic; larger lesions may present with intestinal obstruction, torsion, intussusception, etc. Imaging shows a well-defined echogenic lesion with fon sonography or fat density/intensity lesion with a few thin septa on CT/MRI. Intussusception results in bowel within bowel configuration along with mesenteric fat and vessels within. CT scan is an investigation of choice as it depicts the site, level of intestinal obstruction, transition zone, cause of obstruction, and its complications.

Pitfalls

■ Sonography is an operator-dependent technique and may be missed, especially in obese persons.

Differential Diagnosis

Liposarcoma (thick, nodular septa)

Management

For large tumors, surgery is required.

Case 52 Epiploic Appendagitis

A 38-year-old female with left lower quadrant pain (Figure 2.15).

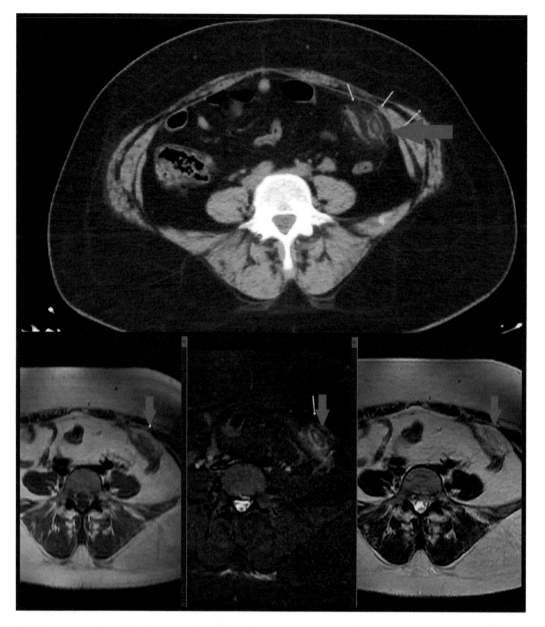

Figure 2.15 CT abdomen shows severe fat stranding and fatty ovoid mass with a hyperattenuated rim in the left lower quadrant. MRI depicts a fat-signal intensity lesion with adjacent stranding on all the sequences.

Discussion

Epiploic appendagitis, a rare self-limited ischemic/inflammatory entity with intraperitoneal focal fat infarction, affects the appendices epiploicae. Patients may be asymptomatic or present with abdominal pain and guarding in a few cases.

Sonography reveals an oval, non-compressible avascular 2–4 cm hyperechoic mass surrounded by hypoechoic stranding. CECT shows a fat density ovoid lesion with a hyperdense rim (hyperdense rim sign), mild fluid collection, and surrounding inflammatory fat stranding. The central hyperdense dot represents a thrombosed vascular pedicle (central dot sign). The lesion is hyperintense (less than normal fat) on T1WI and loss of signal on fat-suppressed T2WI. The thin peripheral rim is hypointense on T1WI, hyperintense on T2WI, and enhances on contrast scans. The central vein is hypointense on T1- and T2WI.

Differential Diagnosis

- Mesenteric panniculitis
- Omental infarction and appendicitis (right-sided usually)
- Diverticulitis

Management

Self-limited

Case 53 Sigmoid Adenocarcinoma with Bowel Perforation and Colo-Vesical Fistula
A 65-year-old female presented with abdominal pain, altered bowel habits, and weight loss (Figure 2.16).

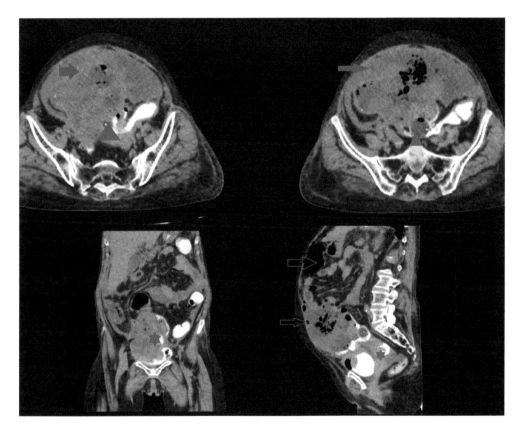

Figure 2.16 CT with positive contrast through Foley's catheter—Asymmetric circumferential heterogeneously enhancing irregular mural thickening (star) involving the sigmoid colon, with adjacent mesocolonic fat stranding, seen infiltrating the dome of the urinary bladder with air foci and contrast opacification (arrowhead) within the bladder. Gross hypodense collection (solid arrow) in the pelvic and peritoneal cavity with numerous air attenuation foci (open arrow) along the peri hepatic, paracolic, and anterior abdominal wall region communicating with the sigmoid colon.

Discussion

Colovesical fistula is an abnormal communication between the colon and bladder resulting in pneumaturia, fecaluria, and recurrent UTIs. The common causes include diverticulitis, malignancy, inflammatory bowel disease, radiotherapy, etc.

Hyperechoic air foci are seen in the non-dependent part of the urinary bladder, along with an irregularly thickened sigmoid colon on sonography. MRI better delineates fistulous communication owing to its inherent soft tissue contrast.

Management

Surgery or palliative treatment such as stenting

APPENDIX

Case 54 Acute Appendicitis

A 32-year-old male presented with RLQ pain, fever, loss of appetite, nausea, and leukocytosis (Figure 2.17).

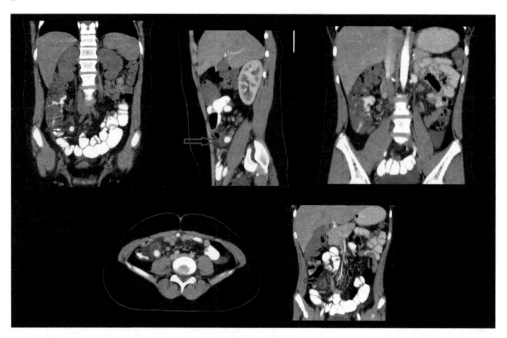

Figure 2.17 NCCT and CECT abdomen depicts a dilated appendix with a thickened, enhancing wall, adjacent fat stranding, and appendicolith (open arrow) with a few small reactive lymph nodes (solid arrow).

Discussion

A normal appendix is an air-filled blind-ending tubular structure with a diameter<7mm that lies medial to the caecum. Typically, it is low to intermediate SI on T2WI. An appendix is a blind-ending tubular structure, and its luminal obstruction due to appendicolith, fecolith, foreign body, ascariasis, or lymphoid hyperplasia results in closed-loop obstruction, distension, inflammation, and bacterial infection, rendering acute appendicitis one of the most frequent causes of abdominal surgery.

Sonography depicts tender, non-compressible, dilated>6mm, blind-ending tubular structure with wall hyperemia, adjacent fluid collection, reactive mesenteric lymphadenopathy usually, and appendicolith sometimes. CECT abdomen reveals stratified hyper-enhancing wall thickening, adjacent inflammatory fat stranding (mild/moderate/severe), reactive lymphadenopathy, appendicolith, and lack of contrast in the appendicular lumen. Wall discontinuity and the presence of free fluid are indicative of perforation. It may be a/w caecal wall thickening and arrowhead sign (funneling of contrast in the cecum centering about obstructed appendicular lumen). Complications such as abscess formation and wall necrosis with subsequent perforation can be delineated well on CECT. Postoperative adhesions may result in SBO.

Differential Diagnosis

- Amebic colitis (circumferential, homogeneously enhancing mural thickening of the terminal ileum and cecum with adjacent adenopathy and relevant history along with normal appendix)

- Ileocecal TB (circumferential wall thickening of the terminal ileum, IC valve, and cecum, along with peripherally enhancing necrotic lymphadenopathy)

- Typhilitis (immunocompromised patients with circumferential and symmetric wall thickening of the cecum and ascending colon)

- Meckel's diverticulitis (located on the antimesenteric border, approximately 100 cm from the ileocecal valve)

- Mesenteric adenitis (right-sided mesenteric lymphadenopathy without an identifiable inflammatory condition)

- Gynecological pathologies (ectopic pregnancy, PID, complicated ovarian cyst)

- Crohn's disease (eccentric wall thickening, mucosal hyperenhancement, engorged vasa recta penetrating the bowel wall—comb sign), fibrofatty proliferation along the mesenteric side of the affected bowel—creeping fat sign)

Atypical locations of the appendix, as in the retrocecal area, within the inguinal canal known as Amyand hernia or within the femoral canal, may result in non-localization of the inflamed appendix.

Management

- Laparoscopic appendectomy for uncomplicated acute appendicitis.

- Initial conservative treatment, depending on the clinical and imaging findings.

Case 55 Appendiceal Abscess

A 48-year-old male presents with abdominal pain and fever (Figure 2.18).

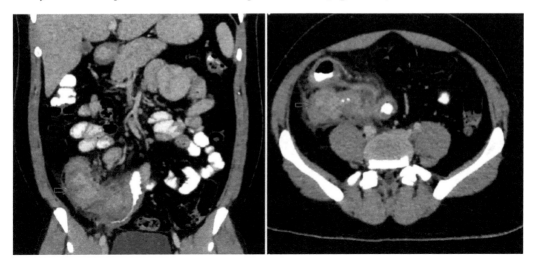

Figure 2.18 CECT abdomen revealed marked circumferential appendicular wall thickening extending into the cecum, IC junction, and terminal ileum, along with adjacent fat stranding, minimal fluid, and reactive mesenteric lymphadenopathy.

Discussion

Inadequately treated appendicitis may get complicated to an appendicular lump characterized by an inflamed appendix and its spread to the adjacent intestine and omentum, forming a localized mass in the RLQ 3–5 days after acute appendicitis. Direct visualization of the appendix may not be possible in an abscess.

Differential Diagnosis

- Appendicular adenocarcinoma (ill-defined peripherally enhancing hypodense lesions with nodular, asymmetric mural thickening of ileum, cecum, and IC junction in elderly)

- Ileocecal TB

- Colitis

- Tubovarian cysts/masses
- Intussusception (bowel within bowel configuration)
- Crohn's disease
- Ectopic kidney
- Psoas abscess

Management

Percutaneous abscess drainage and delayed appendicectomy.

RECTUM AND ANUS

Case 56 Adenocarcinoma of the Rectum with Liver Metastasis

A 69-year-old male presented with alteration in bowel habits and weight loss (Figure 2.19).

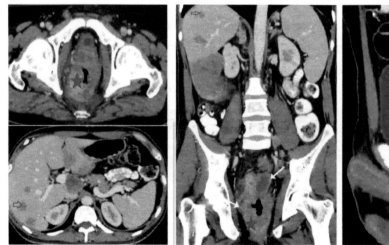
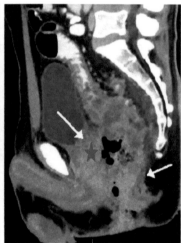

Figure 2.19   CECT abdomen revealed long segment asymmetrical circumferential heterogeneously enhancing thickening causing luminal narrowing of the anorectal region and extending up to the anal verge. The thickening is a/w adjacent fat stranding, regional lymphadenopathy, and prostate and bladder neck infiltration. Multiple heterogeneously enhancing hypodense lesions of varying sizes are noted in the liver.

Discussion

Adenocarcinoma is the most common form of rectal cancer, with most cancers developing from polyps and a higher incidence in the western male population above 60 years, where it is routinely recommended to have regular diagnostic and screening colonoscopy. Patients with Familial Adenomatous polyposis and Lynch Syndrome have a genetic predisposition to rectal cancer. Patients present with abdominal pain, distention, and weakness. Rectal bleeding, alterations in bowel habits, and weight loss often point toward more serious diseases. The lesions can be polypoidal, ulcerating, semi-annular, or annular. Common complications of rectal cancer include bowel obstruction in high-grade tumors, ischemia, hemorrhage, and distant metastasis to the liver, lungs, bones, etc. The prognosis depends upon the extent of adjacent or distant infiltration by the tumor.

Double-contrast barium enema (DCBE), though not used frequently these days, shows filling defects or polypoidal lesions, flat plaques or semi-annular lesions, shouldering or strictures.

Endorectal ultrasonography using flexible probes helps in accurately diagnosing rectal cancer, local invasion, internal and external anal sphincter involvement, and metastasis.

CT scans show the size and extent of mass with asymmetrical wall thickening. TNM staging can be easily done with the help of CT imaging. However, smaller polyps or flat plaque-like lesions are easy to miss on conventional CT. CT colonography may be better suited for such lesions under proper preparation. Tumors are T1 hypointense and T2 hyperintense, though mucinous tumors appear T2 hyperintense. MRI staging of rectal cancer is done considering the circumferential extent of the tumor, presence of lymph nodes, and invasion of the adjacent urinary bladder, uterus, and prostate. The tumor can be low (0–5 cm), mid (5–10 cm), or high (10–15 cm), depending on the distance from the anal verge.

Differential Diagnosis

Rectal carcinoma has to be differentiated from diverticular disease. On imaging, the presence of polyps, shouldering, and straightening of folds favors the diagnosis of carcinoma.

Pitfalls

- A low residue diet and administration of purgative agents such as magnesium sulfate or bisacodyl prior to the exam.
- Residual fecal matter can be tagged with barium sulfate ingested to distinguish it from any mass lesion.
- Smooth muscle relaxation is achieved by administering scopolamine butyl or glucagon intravenously.
- Automatic CO_2 insufflators must be used to properly distend the colon as lesions may be missed in a collapsed colon.
- Prone scans should also be obtained.
- MRI imaging does not require such strict use of purgative agents or colonic distention.

Management

- Almost all cases of rectal carcinoma aim for total mesorectal excision along with chemo and radiotherapy, with circumferential resection margin (CRM) being a good predictor of resection.
- In a few patients with tumors<3 cm situated within 8 cm of the anal verge, transanal microsurgery may be performed.

Liver metastasis was discussed in Chapter 1.

Case 57 Mucinous Rectal Adenocarcinoma

A 27-year-old male with biopsy-proven case (Figure 2.20).

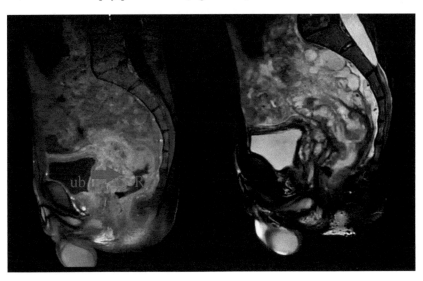

Figure 2.20   MR pelvis shows circumferential irregular polypoidal T1 isointense, T2 heterogenous hyperintense lesion showing mild post-contrast enhancement, causing significant luminal narrowing with mesorectal fat stranding and lobulated T1 isointense, T2 hyperintense cystic components in mesorectum.

Discussion

The mucinous type of rectal adenocarcinoma is a rare histological type; ill-differentiated tumors are usually a/w young age, progressing tumor, high metastatic rates, and poor clinical outcome. On imaging, the tumor shows marked wall thickening with calcium deposition, hyperintense signal intensity on T2WI (due to extracellular mucin), less enhancement, and minimal restriction on DWI. Histopathology report revealed extracellular mucinous material with epithelial cells, eosinophilic cytoplasm, and fibrous stroma and confirmed mucinous carcinoma of the rectum.

Differential Diagnosis

- Response to neoadjuvant treatment due to mucinous degeneration.
- Mucinous metastasis/lymphadenopathy.

Management

Preoperative radiotherapy, surgery, and adjuvant chemotherapy.

Case 58 Perianal Fistula

A 29-year-old patient with pain and pruritis in the anal region (Figure 2.21).

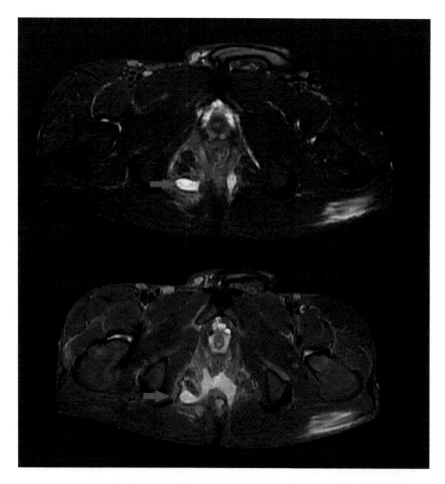

Figure 2.21 MRI pelvis depicts a curvilinear fistulous tract hypointense on T1WI and hyperintense on T2WI and STIR with external opening at 7′0 clock and internal opening at 7–8′0 clock position. Small collection is seen in the right ischioanal region with a horseshoe-shaped extension to the left side. Moderate inflammation and edema are seen around the fistulous tract.

Discussion

Perianal fistulas due to anal gland obstruction are seen commonly in clinical settings, the usual etiologies being tuberculosis, Crohn's disease, trauma, radiation therapy, etc. MRI is done routinely, and fistulas without fibrosis appear hyperintense on T2WI with enhancement. Fistulas can be simple linear or form secondary fistulous tracts with abscess formation. Fistulas are classified as high or low depending on the location of the internal opening relative to the anorectal ring.

Type of fistulas (Table 2.8)

Table 2.8: Types of Anal Fistulas

Intersphincteric (40%–50%)	The tract lies between IAS and EAS Do not cross the EAS
Transsphincteric (20%–25%)	Crosses into ischiorectal space after crossing through the EAS
Suprasphincteric	Crosses superiorly over the puborectalis muscles to reach the skin
Extrasphincteric	Lies outside the EAS

Differential Diagnosis

- Pilonidal sinus pathology
- Proctitis

Management

- Fistulotomy and fistulectomy
- Seton technique (Ksharsutra in Ayurveda)

MISCELLANEOUS

Case 59 Cavitating Mesenteric Lymph Node Syndrome

A 48-year-old male, k/c/o celiac disease, presented with diarrhea, weight loss, and abdominal pain for 4–5 months (Figure 2.22).

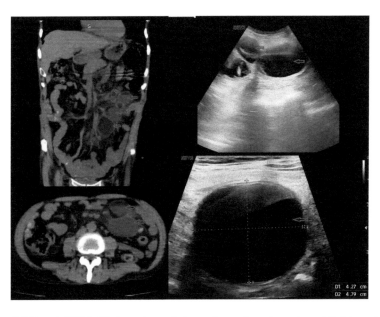

Figure 2.22   USG and CT Multiple, enlarged, hypodense lymph nodes with fat-containing areas and some with fat-fluid levels in the mesentery.

Discussion

Cavitating Mesenteric Lymph Node Syndrome (CMLNS) is a rare complication of celiac disease with clinical presentation as diarrhea, steatorrhea, fatigue, weight loss, and abdominal pain, and the radiological triad of cavitation mesenteric lymph nodes with fat-fluid levels, splenic atrophy and villous atrophy on upper UGI endoscopic biopsy. Extraintestinal manifestations include anemia, osteopenia, aphthous ulcers, peripheral neuropathy, dementia, seizures, and dermatitis herpetiformis. Sonography may show dilated bowel, increased peristalsis, and thickened bowel wall. T2WI and T1WI show fat-fluid levels in the lymph nodes. Patient with celiac disease is at high risk of developing T-cell lymphoma with the involvement of multiple lymph node groups without fat content along with splenomegaly. FNAC reveals milky fluid from the lymph nodes.

Differential Diagnosis

Though cavitary mesenteric lymph nodes with fat-fluid levels and splenic atrophy are characteristic of CMLNS, other causes of hypoattenuating lymph nodes are tuberculosis, Whipple's disease, necrotic metastases, germ cell tumors, and lymphoma. However, these causes involve multiple nodal groups and cause splenomegaly.

Management

Strict gluten-free diet.

Case 60 Omental Infarct

A 56-year-old female presented with severe and intermittent RUQ pain with nonspecific symptoms of nausea (Figure 2.23).

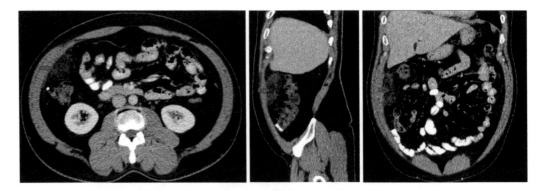

Figure 2.23 CECT abdomen depicts a well-circumscribed area with inflammation centered around the omental fat.

Discussion

Omentum is a vascular-rich peritoneal fold with abundant collaterals. Hence, omental infarction is a rare self-limited entity resulting in fat necrosis due to interruption of its blood supply, presenting with acute abdominal pain (RLQ frequently) and nonspecific symptoms. They are mostly a/w obesity, abdominal trauma, and surgery.

It presents as an ill-defined area of fat stranding in the early course and later becomes a relatively well-defined focal heterogenous mass with fat stranding between the anterior abdominal wall and colon. Disproportionate fat stranding without bowel wall thickening helps differentiate it from adjacent familiar pathological entities. Fat components are reduced in the chronic stages. On sonography, it is noted as a fixed, echogenic, non-compressible, tender mass in the omentum with reduced or absent flow. Omental infarcts are FDG avid and simulate tumors if not correlated with CT findings.

Differential Diagnosis

1. *Appendicitis*: Bowel wall thickening a/w fat stranding

2. *Epiploic Appendagitis*: Thrombosed vessel gives central dot sign

3. Diverticulitis

4. Tumors like liposarcoma grow over time, and so do not present with acute abdominal pain.

Management

- Conservative treatment with anti-inflammatory, prophylactic antibiotics, and analgesic drugs.

- Surgery, only if operable.

Case 61 Body Packer

A 27-year-old male caught at the airport (Figure 2.24).

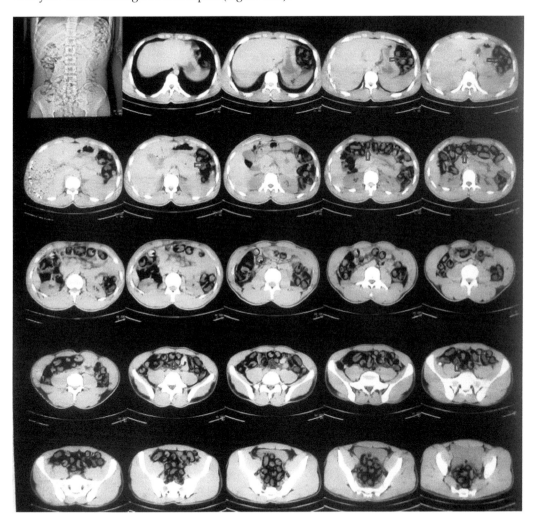

Figure 2.24 CT abdomen depicting multiple, round to oval hypo to isodense foreign bodies surrounded by a gas halo.

Discussion

One of the most popular methods for smuggling illegal substances is body packing/stuffing by drug mules, who insert or swallow drugs, such as cocaine, cannabis, and heroin, through the gastrointestinal system or other openings. These packets, if isodense, can be identified on radiographs.

Plain X-ray and CT show multiple, well-defined, round to oval, low-density foreign bodies surrounded by a gas halo in the stomach, small and large bowel. CT differentiates between a variety of drugs depending on their HU—cocaine, less dense than fat (–220 HU), cannabis (simulates bone 700 HU), and heroin (–500 HU, between fat and air).

Complications, such as intestinal obstruction, perforation, and peritonitis, may occur due to drug packets or drug toxicity due to packet rupture.

Management

- *Asymptomatic Cases*: Laxatives

- *Symptomatic Patients*: Surgery

PEDIATRIC

Case 62 Congenital Hypertrophic Pyloric Stenosis

A 6-week-old neonate with vomiting (Figure 2.25).

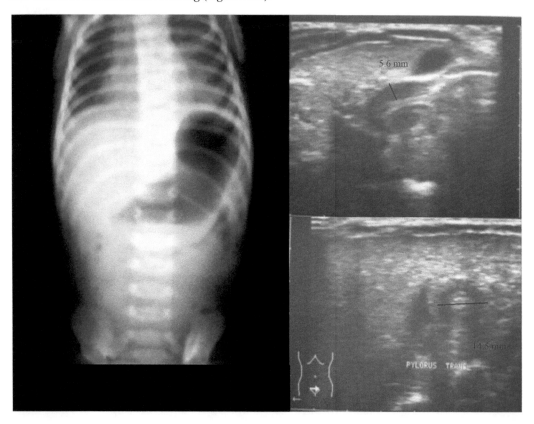

Figure 2.25 Abdominal X-ray shows a distended stomach with minimal distal intestinal bowel gas. Sonography depicts a hypoechoic hypertrophied pyloric wall of 5.6 mm thickness, the pyloric canal measuring 17.5 mm in length (cervix sign), and includes hyperechoic central mucosa in transverse diameter measuring 14.5 mm (target sign), validating pyloric hypertrophy.

Discussion

Hypertrophic pyloric stenosis (HPS), the idiopathic thickening (both hyperplasia and hypertrophy) of circular muscle fibers of gastric pyloric antral musculature, leading to GOO, is common in firstborn, bottle-fed males who were delivered through cesarean section.

The infant presents with non-bilious projectile vomiting, palpable mass, and hypochloremic metabolic alkalosis.

Barium meal shows delayed gastric emptying, elongated pylorus with a narrow lumen (string-sign), beak-shaped pyloric antrum. Sonography shows hypoechoic hypertrophied muscle and hyperechoic central mucosa with dimensions of single muscular wall > 3 mm, pyloric length > 15 mm (cervix sign), and pyloric transverse diameter > 13 mm (target sign).

Management

- Rehydration and electrolyte imbalance correction

- Pyloromyotomy

Case 63 Malrotation with Midgut Volvulus

A severely malnourished three-year-old boy presented with abdominal pain and bilious vomiting for 8–10 days (Figure 2.26).

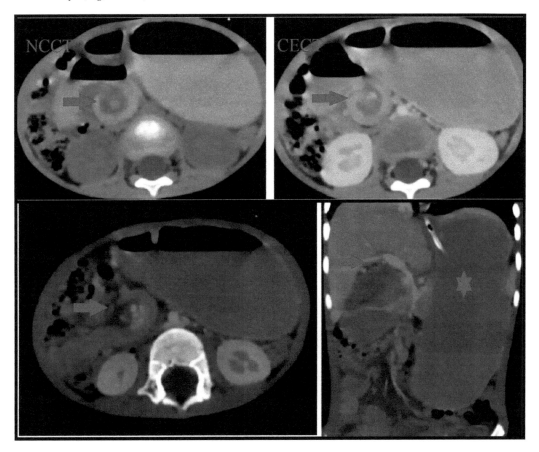

Figure 2.26 Whirlpool appearance (arrow) of small bowel loops and mesentery wrapping (one and half turn) around SMA in the right lumbar region, resulting in dilatation of proximal bowel loops and stomach (star). Normal enhancement of SMV and bowel wall on CECT.

Discussion

Midgut volvulus, an anomaly of rotation and fixation, occurs with the twisting of intestines (malrotation) upon themselves, resulting in the blockage of blood flow. It is more frequent in males, and presentation is with bilious vomiting and failure to thrive. Volvulus generally occurs due to long mesentery/short mesenteric root with abnormal bowel motility. It could be primary or secondary due to anatomical defects, adhesions, ascariasis, tumors, etc.

Usually done in a stable child, the upper gastrointestinal series shows an abnormally placed duodenojejunal junction (DJ) to the right of the vertebral body with dilatation of the proximal bowel and stomach, giving a double-bubble sign. Corkscrew appearance is noted in complete obstruction with the entire small intestine on the right side. Imaging reveals the whirlpool sign with the vessels twisting around the base of the mesentery and an anomalous relation of superior mesenteric vessels with SMV lying anterior and to the left of SMA. It may be complicated as bowel ischemia and necrosis.

Differential Diagnosis

- Other causes of neonatal bowel obstruction, such as duodenal/jejunal atresia, webs, and annular pancreas.

- Ladd bands.

- Extrinsic compression on the duodenum

- Necrotizing enterocolitis

- Neonatal sepsis

- Pyloric stenosis (non-bilious vomiting)

Management

Surgery

Case 64 Hirschsprungs Disease

A full-term male infant presented with abdominal distension and delay in the passage of meconium (Figure 2.27).

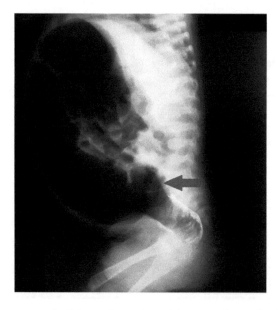

Figure 2.27 Roentgenogram depicts an abrupt transition zone (arrow) with proximal colon dilatation.

Discussion

Hirschsprung's disease, a common cause of low intestinal obstruction, is frequent in male infants and infrequent in premature babies.

Failure of craniocaudal migration of myenteric ganglion cells from the neural crests to intestines between the 7th and 12th weeks of gestation results in the aganglionic segment (rectum is always involved) with proximal dilatation of normal bowel. The normal rectosigmoid ratio in children is > 1, and reversal suggests Hirschsprung's disease.

It can be of four types depending on the aganglionic segment—short (rectum, sigmoid colon), long (up to distal transverse colon), ultrashort (anal sphincter), or total colonic aganglionosis (extension into the small bowel).

Characteristic findings include:

- Transition zone between the aganglionic distal and ganglionic proximal (dilated) segments

- Impaired peristaltic waves resulting in saw-tooth appearance/fasciculations of abnormal segment

- Retention of contrast in delayed films
- Parallel transverse folds in normal colon proximally

Definitive diagnosis is via rectal biopsy.

Differential Diagnosis of Micro Colon

- Meconium ileus
- Small (lazy) left colon syndrome
- MMIHS (Megacystis Microcolon Intestinal Hypoperistalsis Syndrome)
- Colonic atresia

Management

Surgery

Case 65 Ascariasis

A 17-year-old female with abdominal pain and vomiting (Figure 2.28).

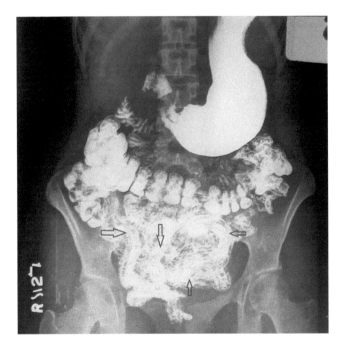

Figure 2.28   Barium study depicts numerous linear tubular filling defects within the small bowel.

Discussion

Ascariasis is among the common helminthic infections encountered, especially in developing countries, transmitted via the fecal-oral route. Ingested eggs hatch in the small bowel and the mucosa is penetrated by larvae, which are transmitted hematogeneously to the hepatobiliary, tracheobronchial tree, etc. It may cause complications, such as cholangitis/biliary colic, intestinal obstruction, appendicitis, pancreatitis, and volvulus/intussusception by a large worm bolus. Loeffler's pneumonia occurs with the migration of worms to the lungs, resulting in eosinophilia and alveolar infiltrates.

Contrast studies show elongated tubular filling defects in the small intestine (inner tube/spaghetti sign in longitudinal section and target/bull's eye in transverse section). Sonography reveals paired echogenic lines separated by an anechoic area in the longitudinal section and an echogenic ring in the transverse section.

Management

Albendazole 400 mg.
Surgery in complicated cases.

Case 66 Meconium Peritonitis

A neonate with abdominal distension (Figure 2.29).

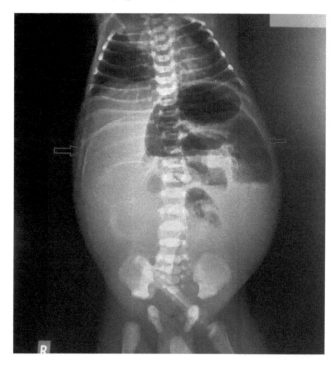

Figure 2.29   Abdominal radiograph showing peripheral calcification of a meconium pseudocyst.

Discussion

In utero intestinal perforation due to bowel atresia or meconium ileus, resulting in meconium leakage into the fetal peritoneal cavity and sterile chemical peritonitis. Ascites, calcification, fibrosis (bowel obstruction), and occasionally the creation of cysts with calcific rim are the outcomes of secondary inflammatory reactions. Usually, the gut is intact at delivery, the perforation seals off, and intraperitoneal meconium calcifies within 24 hours. The calcifications can be linear, curvilinear, or flocculent. Scrotal calcifications are evident if the processus vaginalis is patent. Sonography shows echogenic foci with posterior acoustic shadowing on the peritoneal surface and echogenic ascites, giving a snowstorm appearance.

Management

Isolated calcifications may heal spontaneously. Complicated cases require surgery.

SUGGESTED READINGS

Drake, R. L., & Vogl, A. W. (2020). *Gray's Atlas of Anatomy E-Book*. Elsevier Health Sciences.

Gore, R. M., & Levine, M. S. (2014). *Textbook of Gastrointestinal Radiology E-Book*. Elsevier Health Sciences.

Jaffe, T., & Thompson, W. M., Large-bowel obstruction in the adult: Classic radiographic and CT findings, etiology, and mimics. *Radiology* 2015;275:3, 651–663.

Lumley, J. S., & Craven, J. L. (2018). *Bailey & Love's Essential Clinical Anatomy*. CRC Press.

3 Urinary System

INTRODUCTION

EMBRYOLOGY

The development of the urinary system and reproductive system occurs in conjunction as they share a common genesis from intermediate mesoderm (urogenital ridge), which differentiates into nephrogenic ridge (kidneys, ureter) laterally and gonadal ridge (testes/ovaries) medially.

The kidneys develop in three successive stages in the intermediate mesoderm.

- *Pronephros*: In the cervical region, it is non-functional and regresses completely.

- *Mesonephros*: In the thoracolumbar region, forms ureteric buds in both sexes and genital duct in males with regression in females.

- *Metanephros*: In the sacral region, forms the metanephric blastema.

Each permanent kidney develops from the following:

- Ureteric bud gives rise to the ureter, renal pelvis, calyces, and collecting tubules (mesonephric duct) which form a collecting part.

- Metanephric blastema gives rise to nephrons and develops into excretory parts of the (Figure 3.1).

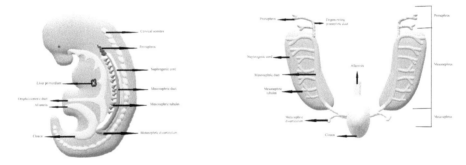

Figure 3.1 Renal embryology.

From the pelvic position (blood supply from common iliac artery branches), the kidney ascends to its final position in the abdomen (with renal branches of the abdominal aorta). The pelvic vessels usually disappear. Initially, the hilum is ventral, then rotates medially at about 90° and becomes medial. The lobulated contour of the fetal kidney disappears at the end of the fetal period. With the kidney's ascent, the ureters elongate and open into the bladder superiorly.

The urinary bladder develops from the endoderm-lined, upper part of the endoderm-lined urogenital sinus, which is continuous with the allantois. The bladder's trigone is formed by the lower part of the mesonephric ducts, which is integrated into the urogenital sinus wall. The connective tissue and smooth muscle that envelop the bladder originate from the adjoining splanchnic mesoderm. The allantois degenerates and persists as the fibrous cord called the urachus or median umbilical ligament.

The anorectal septum divides the cloaca anteriorly into the urogenital sinus (UGS) and posteriorly into the anus. The UGS is divided into the upper part (bladder) and lower part (urethra and female reproductive tract).

Table 3.1 illustrates the male and female derivatives of the urogenital sinus.

Table 3.1: **Male and Female Derivatives of the Urogenital Sinus (UGS)**

	UGS (Pelvic Part)	UGS (Phallic Part)/Urethra Plate
Female	Whole urethra and part of the vagina	Vestibule, labia minora
Male	Prostatic and membranous part	Spongy (bulbar and penile) part

DOI: 10.1201/9781003452034-3

ANATOMY URINARY SYSTEM

The urinary or excretory system consists of kidneys, ureters, urinary bladder, and urethra.

Kidneys

The kidneys are bean-shaped, reddish-brown excretory organs located retroperitoneally on the posterior abdominal wall, one on each side of the vertebral column, opposite T12 and L3. The left kidney lies at a slightly higher level than the right one. The hilum transmits the renal vein, renal artery, and renal pelvis from before backward, along with lymph vessels and sympathetic fibers. The following layers from the inside cover each kidney outwards: fibrous capsule, perirenal fat, renal fascia, and pararenal fat.

Each kidney has a medulla with renal pyramids, whose apex, called the renal papilla, projects medially, and a cortex extending between the pyramids is the renal column of Bertin. The nephrons are located within the cortex. Eight to thirteen pyramids make up the medulla, and they end at the level of the calyces in the renal papillae. The renal sinus is the space within the hilum that contains the renal pelvis. The renal pelvis divides into major and minor calyces.

Each renal artery arises from the aorta at the level of L2. Each artery bifurcates into anterior and posterior divisions, supplying the kidney's apical, upper, middle, lower, and posterior segments. The segmental arteries further divide into lobar artery, interlobar artery, arcuate artery, and interlobular artery till the level of afferent glomerular arterioles. The left and right renal veins drain into the left renal vein and IVC. The kidneys drain into the lateral aortic group of lymph nodes.

Ureter

Each ureter, 25 cm long and 3 mm diameter, is a retroperitoneally located, thick muscular tube with active peristaltic contractions through which urine passes from the renal pelvis to the urinary bladder.

Constrictions in the ureter at different levels

1. At the pelvi-ureteric junction (PUJ)

2. At the brim of the lesser pelvis

3. Point of the crossing of the ureter by ductus deferens or broad ligament

4. Passage through the bladder wall at vesicoureteric junction (VUJ)

5. At its opening in the trigone

It starts at the tip of the transverse process of the L2 vertebra and then follows the line of tips of the transverse processes of the remaining vertebrae. It crosses in front of the sacroiliac joint and then runs along the anterior margin of the greater sciatic notch till it reaches the ischial spine.

The renal artery supplies the upper part of the ureter, the middle portion by the gonadal artery, and the pelvic part by the superior vesical artery, uterine, and middle rectal artery.

Venous blood drains into the corresponding veins. The lymph drains into the lateral aortic and iliac group of lymph nodes.

Urinary Bladder

The urinary bladder, a hollow muscular organ, acts as a temporary urine reservoir. When the bladder becomes sufficiently distended to sense the urge to micturate, the stored urine escapes through the urethra. It varies in shape, size, and position according to its urine content. It lies entirely within the pelvis when empty (tetrahedral shape) and extends upwards into the abdominal cavity when full (ovoid shape), reaching the umbilicus or higher.

The mucous membrane of the greater part of the empty bladder is thrown into folds that disappear when full. The area of the membrane covering the internal surface of the base of the bladder is called trigone. The mucous membrane is firmly adherent to the underlying muscle coat, which is always smooth even when the bladder is empty. The superior angle of the trigone corresponds to the opening of the ureter and the inferior angle to the internal urethral orifice. The interureteric muscular ridge extends between the openings of the ureter.

True ligaments are the condensation of pelvic fascia around the neck and the base of the bladder and include the lateral true ligament, posterior ligament, and medial and lateral puboprostatic/pubovesical ligament of the bladder. False ligaments are peritoneal folds, which do not form any support to the bladder and include median, medial, and lateral umbilical ligaments.

- *Blood Supply*: Vesical arteries, branches of the anterior trunk of the internal iliac artery. The veins form the vesical venous plexus and drain into the internal iliac vein.

- *Lymphatic Drainage*: External and internal iliac nodes.

Urethra

It is a tubular channel through which urine and seminal fluid pass in males and only urine in females.

Male Urethra

The male urethra, about 18–20 cm long, extends from the internal urethral orifice (neck of the urinary bladder) to the external urethral orifice (tip of the glans penis).

Parts of Male Urethra

According to its location, the urethra has the following parts:

a. Preprostatic part extends from the bladder neck to the base of the prostate.

b. Prostatic part (passes through the prostate) is 3 cm long, horseshoe-shaped in cross-section, and is the most dilatable and the widest part of the male urethra. It has the prostatic utricle, ejaculatory ducts, and prostatic gland openings.

c. Membranous part (passes through the urogenital diaphragm) is 1.5–2 cm long and is the narrowest and least dilatable part. It is star-shaped in cross-section. Minute mucous glands open into it.

d. Spongy or penile part (passes through the corpus spongiosum of the penis) is 15 cm long and is mostly uniform in diameter with medium dilations. Urethral or Littre's glands open into it. In cross-section, its shape varies from trapezoid, transverse slit to vertical slit from above downwards.

The urethra is supplied by the inferior vesical, middle rectal, and penile branches of internal pudendal arteries. The blood is drained by the prostatic venous plexus, which finally drains into the internal iliac vein.

Lymphatic Drainage: Prostatic and membranous urethra drains into internal iliac lymph nodes and penile urethra into deep inguinal lymph nodes.

Female Urethra

The female urethra, with an average length of 4 cm, is shorter than the male urethra. It extends from the urinary bladder neck to the external urethral meatus in the vaginal vestibule, where the urethral orifice is placed in front of the vaginal orifice and is about 2.5 cm behind the clitoris. In cross-section at different levels, the shape of the female urethra differs from crescentic, star-shaped, transverse slit to sagittal slit. There are several urethral and paraurethral glands (of Skene) along the urethra and pit-like mucous recesses called urethral lacunae. The urethra has an internal and external sphincter.

- The internal sphincter (sphincter vesicae) is involuntary, surrounds the internal urethral orifice, and is formed from the muscle of the bladder wall.

- The external sphincter (sphincter urethrae) is voluntary, surrounds the membranous part of the urethra, and is derived from the sphincter urethrae muscle.

- *Blood Supply*: Branches of superior vesical and vaginal arteries. The internal iliac vein drains the blood.

- *Lymphatic Drainage*: Internal and external iliac nodes.

NORMAL VARIANTS

- *Hypertrophied column of Bertin*

The hypertrophic renal parenchyma extending into the renal sinus has a characteristic conical shape, most frequently noted at the junction of the kidney's upper and middle pole. This entity is isoechoic/dense/intense to the normal renal parenchyma on all imaging modalities.

■ *Dromedary hump*

A localized bulging on the left kidney's lateral contour due to the splenic imprint on the superolateral kidney.

■ *Persistent fetal lobulation*

Smooth indentation of renal contour that may simulate scarring if irregular.

SPECTRUM OF CALCULI IN THE URINARY SYSTEM AND GRADING OF HYDRONEPHROSIS

Case 67 Staghorn Calculus

A 32-year-old male presented with colicky flank pain, hematuria, and difficulty in urination (Figure 3.2).

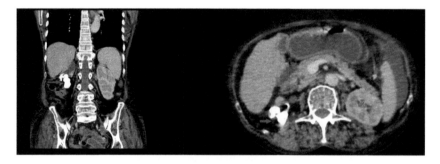

Figure 3.2 CT abdomen depicts irregular-shaped, hyperdense (+ 873 HU) calculus in the right renal pelvis leading to moderate hydronephrosis and cortical thinning of mildly atrophic (6.9 * 4.2 cm) right kidney. The note is made of perisplenic and perihepatic collections in a cirrhotic liver.

Discussion

Nephro/urolithiasis, calcific foci in the renal collecting system, are frequently encountered in routine practice. Magnesium ammonium phosphate (MAP) or struvite calculi take the branching shape of the renal pelvis and calyces and simulate the horns of a stag. They are common due to recurrent infection due to urease-producing bacteria such as Proteus, Klebsiella, etc.

Table 3.2 depicts the anatomical site of calculus and the region of pain it produces.

Table 3.2: Anatomical Site of Renal Calculus and the Region of Pain It Produces

Calculus	Location of Pain
Renal pelvis, proximal ureter	Flank
Distal ureter	Pain radiating to the groin region
Ureterovesical junction	Urinary urgency, suprapubic discomfort

Calculi may be asymptomatic and detected incidentally. Apart from pain, calculi present with features of obstruction, and superimposed infection may lead to sepsis mandating urinary decompression.

X-ray kidney ureter bladder (KUB) shows a laminated, radiopaque branching lesion. Calcium, oxalate, and MAP calculi are radiopaque compared to uric acid and cysteine calculi, which are radiolucent. Sonography reveals a densely echogenic (calcified) and branching lesion with posterior acoustic shadowing. Color Doppler may show twinkling artifacts due to stone. CT scans with low-dose protocol (with automated tube current modulation) and iterative image reconstructions are commonly used. MRI shows calculus as signal void on both T1 and T2 WI. Dual Energy CT (DECT) uses high and low voltages to compare the density of different materials to determine stone composition and can also create virtually enhanced images.

It is essential to mention the number, size, and anatomic localization. Additional consideration should be given to stones impacted at the ureteropelvic junction (UPJ), ureter passage over the pelvic brim, and ureterovesical junction (UVJ).

Management

- Most calculi (<5 mm) pass spontaneously.

- Percutaneous nephrolithotomy and extracorporeal shock wave lithotripsy (ESWL) are the preferred treatment for larger stones.

Hydronephrosis

Hydronephrosis refers to pelvicalyceal system (PCS) dilatation due to obstruction (renal/ureteric calculi or other structural/functional pathologies). Calculi>5 mm may get impacted at various constrictions, though <4 mm calculi pass into the bladder naturally. Patients present with flank pain, dysuria, urinary urgency, etc.

Grades of hydronephrosis, depending on PCS dilatation (Table 3.3)

Table 3.3: Grades of Hydronephrosis, Depending on PCS Dilatation

I	Minimal PCS splitting
II	Mildly dilatation
III	Moderate dilatation+mild parenchymal atrophy
IV	Marked dilatation+severe parenchymal thinning

Differential Diagnosis

- Cysts do not communicate with a dilated calyceal system.

- Overfilled bladder relaxes after micturition, and hydronephrosis disappears

Management

Depending on the cause and severity

Case 68 Distal Left Ureteric Calculus with CKD

A 30-year-old patient with flank pain and dysuria (Figure 3.3).

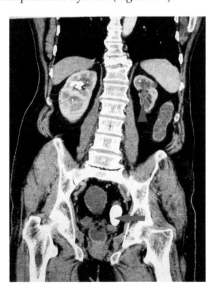

Figure 3.3 Depicts distal left ureteric calculus (arrow) near VUJ, with a small and contracted left kidney (arrowhead) with thinned-out renal parenchyma and a small hyperdense calculus at the upper pole. Multiple right renal calculi with mild hydronephrosis.

Discussion

On X-ray, ureteral calculi should be differentiated from phleboliths (insignificant rounded vascular calcifications with a lucent center).

Discussed in Case 1

Case 69 Vesicouretric Junction Calculus

A 42 year-old male with urinary urgency and pain RLQ (Figure 3.4).

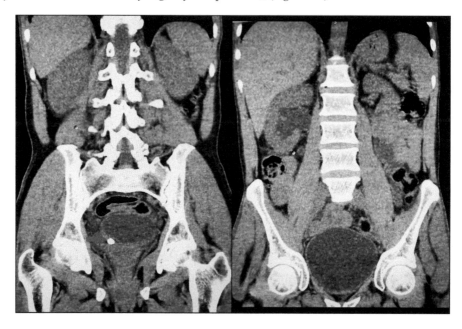

Figure 3.4 CECT abdomen depicts obstructing right VUJ calculus (arrow) with mild-moderate hydronephrosis (star).

Case 70 Moderate Hydronephrosis

A 38-year-old patient with flank pain and urinary urgency (Figure 3.5).

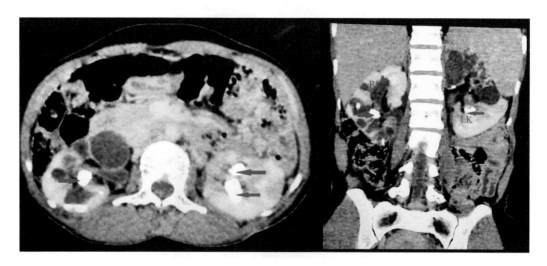

Figure 3.5 CECT abdomen depicts multiple bilateral renal calculi with moderate to severe hydronephrosis and parenchymal thinning.

Case 71 Severe Hydroureteronephrosis

A 40-year-old patient with severe abdominal discomfort (Figure 3.6).

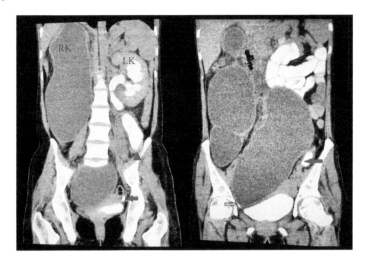

Figure 3.6 CT urography depicts marked dilatation of right PCS with paper thinning of renal parenchyma and markedly dilated right ureter completely occupying abdominopelvic cavity due to distal ureteric stricture causing minimal retrograde filling (open arrow) of contrast from the bladder. No contrast excretion was noted in the right kidney, even in the delayed films. Moderate dilatation of left PCS and proximal to mid ureter with partial stricture (mildly thickened ureteric wall and periureteric fat stranding-arrowhead). Normally excreting left kidney.

Case 72 Encrusted DJ Stent

A 27-year-old female with a forgotten DJ stent (Figure 3.7).

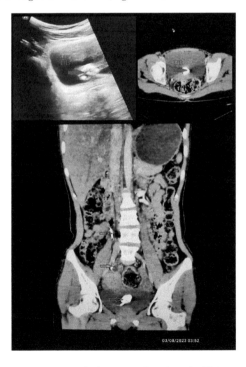

Figure 3.7 The encrusted (peri-stent calcification) distal end of DJ stent in the urinary bladder lumen and normal proximal end in the renal pelvis (no dislodgement of stent).

Discussion

Ureteral stents are inserted to reduce urinary obstruction and aid drainage into the urinary bladder. Complications such as infection, encrustation, misplacement, fragmentation, and migration may occur with prolonged time and forgotten stents, mainly due to a lack of awareness and irregular follow-ups. The patient may present with irritative voiding symptoms, hematuria, flank pain.

Encrustation refers to the adherence of mineral crystals on the stent surface and lumen, especially in forgotten/retained stents. Mineral deposition results in a calcified and brittle stent with susceptibility to stent fracture and ureter avulsion during extraction, increasing the likelihood of developing CKD and necessitating hospitalization for sepsis or UTIs.

Be Cautious

- Take care to remove the distal end first.

- Ensure patient counseling post-DJ-stenting.

Management

- *Mild Encrustation*: Stent extraction using a cystoscope.

- *Moderate*: ESWL, transurethral cystolithotomy, ureteroscopy, and PCNL.

- *Severe*: percutaneous nephrostomy with antibiotics/nephrectomy.

- Newer stents (silicone-based) should be used.

Case 73 Renal Sinus Lipomatosis

A 60-year-old female for routine scan (Sonography revealed enlarged echogenic sinuses with atrophic kidneys) (Figure 3.8).

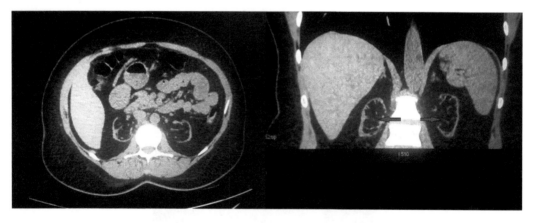

Figure 3.8 NCCT abdomen depicts enlarged sinus fat in bilateral kidneys associated with atrophy of the renal parenchyma.

Discussion

The chronic degenerative process with replacement of renal sinuses by fatty tissue is usually due to aging, calculi, chronic inflammation, transplant kidney, increased exogenous administration, or endogenous production of steroids. It is sometimes used interchangeably with renal replacement lipomatosis, which is the severe form with fat proliferation in the renal sinus and perinephric space with marked destruction/atrophy of renal parenchyma, often a/w XGP. Sonography shows enlarged echogenic central sinuses due to replacement by fat, and CT/MRI can corroborate the findings.

Differential Diagnosis

Fat-containing renal tumors such as renal lipoma, AML, etc.

Management

Observation

Case 74 Polycystic Kidney Disease

A 20-year-old patient with abdominal mass and hematuria (Figure 3.9).

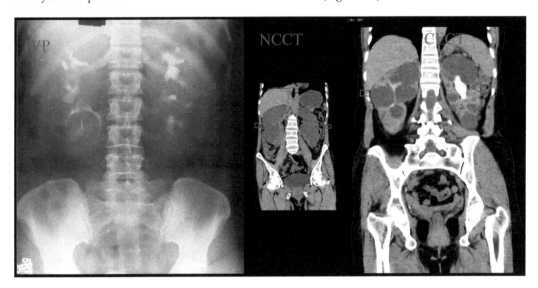

Figure 3.9 IVP depicts a spider-leg appearance. CT reveals multiple renal cysts of varying sizes involving the cortex and medulla of bilaterally enlarged kidneys.

Discussion

PCKD is a hereditary disease with renal architectural distortion, which may be asymptomatic or may present with flank mass, hypertension, hematuria, and progressively impaired renal function. It is usually a/w extrarenal complications such as cysts in the liver, spleen, pancreas, lungs, and seminal vesicles, cerebral Berry aneurysms, heart diseases, aortic dissection, diverticular disease, etc. It may be present in children as the spectrum of ARPCKD ranges from being asymptomatic to severe disease.

Imaging shows bilaterally enlarged, lobulated kidneys with multiple cysts, which increase in size and number with age, along with propensity of infections, hemorrhage, calculi, rupture, malignancy, and end-stage renal failure. IVP shows a spider-leg appearance on the pyelogram due to stretching and distortion of the PCS. A striated nephrogram with radiating dilated collecting ducts may be seen in ARPCKD bilaterally. Sonography depicts the appearance of Swiss cheese due to multiple smoothly marginated cysts of varying sizes involving both the cortex and medulla. Kidneys appear echogenic when cysts are small in size. High-resolution T2WI depicts hyperintense cysts. PCKD may be unilateral in some cases.

Differential Diagnosis

- Acquired cystic diseases of kidneys due to dialysis, etc.
- Multicystic dysplastic kidney
- Medullary cystic disease

Management

- Supportive treatment
- Renal transplantation

Case 75 Medullary Nephrocalcinosis

A 45-year-old patient with hyperparathyroidism presents with flank pain (Figure 3.10).

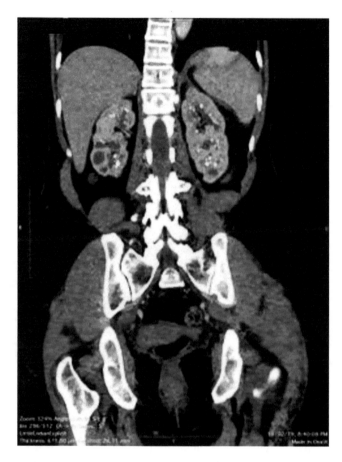

Figure 3.10 Amorphous, coarse calcification in bilateral medullary pyramids (nephrocalcinosis).

Discussion

Medullary nephrocalcinosis, the calcification in the renal parenchyma, is more common than cortical nephrocalcinosis due to the concentrating effects of Henle's loop, which lie in the renal medulla. Calcium nodules rupture into the calyceal system to become urinary stones and may present with renal colic, UTI, and hematuria.

Table 3.4 discusses the differences between the two types of nephrocalcinosis

Table 3.4: **Types of Nephrocalcinosis**

Medullary	Cortical
Medullary sponge kidney, hyperparathyroidism, and renal tubular acidosis	Acute cortical necrosis, chronic glomerulonephritis, and oxalosis
Bilateral stippled calcification in medullary pyramids (central)	Thin peripheral band of calcification

Differential Diagnosis

Punctate, amorphous parenchymal calcifications of renal amyloidosis

Management

Hydration
  Dietary modification with the use of citrates

Case 76 Xanthogranulomatous Pyelonephritis (XGP)

A 56-year-old male with urinary complaints (Figure 3.11).

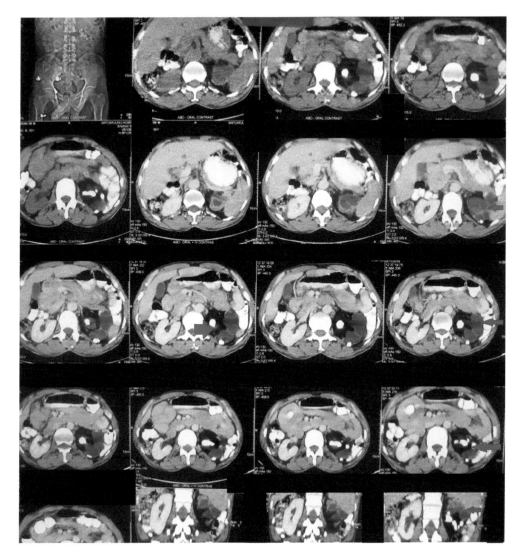

Figure 3.11 CECT abdomen reveals a staghorn calculus in a non-functioning left kidney with interspersed fatty areas.

Discussion

Xanthogranulomatous pyelonephritis (XGP) is a chronic granulomatous infection common in elderly females and diabetics due to *E. coli* or Proteus mirabilis infection and a/w staghorn calculus. It is characterized by the destruction of renal parenchyma and the replacement of normal renal architecture with hypodense lesions filled with pus, debris, and lipid-laden foamy macrophages. Few fat attenuation areas may be seen within the lesion. Three stages of XGP are:

a. Localized to the kidney

b. Gerota's fascia extension

c. Pararenal and retroperitoneal involvement

Differential Diagnosis

- Necrotic RCC
- Pyogenic/tubercular renal abscess
- Emphysematous pyelonephritis

Management

Surgery

Case 77 Emphysematous Pyelonephritis

Case: A 59-year-old diabetic female presented with fever and flank pain (Figure 3.12).

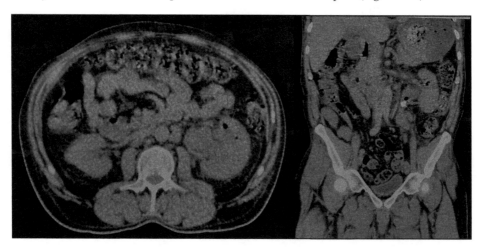

Figure 3.12   NCCT abdomen reveals mildly enlarged left kidney with few air attenuation foci (open arrows) in proximal ureter, upper and mid pole of left kidney with perinephric stranding and thickened Zuckerandl's and lateral conal fascia. Left proximal ureteric calculus (solid arrow) with upstream moderate hydroureteronephrosis (star)—Type 2 EPN.

Discussion

EPN represents necrotizing infection by gas-forming bacteria (*E. coli*, Proteus mirabilis) of renal parenchyma, collecting system, and perirenal tissues, common in females, diabetics, and immuno-compromised patients.

Table 3.5 depicts the stages of EPN.

Table 3.5: Stages of Emphysematous Pyelonephritis

Stage	Findings	Management
1	Gas in the unilateral collecting system only	Parenteral fluids and antibiotics, electrolytes, and glucose control
2	Gas in the unilateral renal parenchyma only	Antibiotics, percutaneous catheter drainage (PCD)
3	Gas in unilateral perinephric/pararenal space	Antibiotics, drainage, and nephrectomy (if risk factors are present)
4	Bilateral kidneys involvement	Antibiotics, drainage, and nephrectomy (if risk factors are present)

Table 3.6 differentiates between two types of EPN.

Table 3.6: Types of Emphysematous Pyelonephritis

Type	EPN 1	EPN 2
Renal parenchymal destruction	>⅓	<⅓
Pattern of gas	Streaky/mottled	Bubbly/loculated
Renal/perirenal fluid collections	Absent	Present
Gas in the collecting system/ureter	Not necessarily	May be seen
Prognosis	Aggressive/worse prognosis	Favorable

Sonography reveals an enlarged kidney with echogenic foci that give reverberation artifacts/ dirty shadowing. It must be differentiated from renal calculi and necrotizing psoas abscess on sonography. CT is confirmatory and also delineates the extent of the disease. Signal void is noted on T1- and T2WI of MRI.

Differential diagnosis

■ Instrumentation/intervention in the urinary tract

■ Fistulous communication with bowel

■ Emphysematous pyelitis (gas in the collecting system, not in the parenchyma)

Management

■ Drainage with antibiotics

■ Surgery in extensive cases

Case 78 Multifocal Acute Pyelonephritis

A 35-year-old patient with flank pain and systemic symptoms (Figure 3.13).

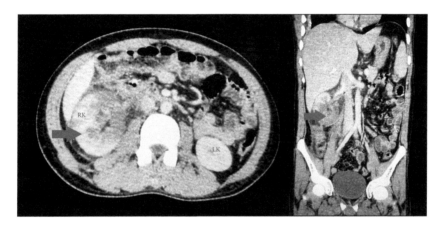

Figure 3.13 CECT abdomen depicts a mildly bulky right kidney with multiple non-enhancing hypodense areas (involving both cortex and medulla) in the mid and lower poles, along with perinephric fat stranding and thickened renal fascias.

Discussion

Acute pyelonephritis, a bacterial infection of renal parenchyma and pelvis, frequently occurs due to ascending infection from the bladder extending to collecting tubules. It is common in females due to short urethra. Patients may present with fever, flank pain, vomiting, urinary urgency, etc.

Sonography may be normal or show localized hypoechoic regions with decreased vascularity on CDUS. CT is better at delineating the hypodense non-enhancing areas extending up to the cortex and evaluating complications such as renal abscesses, chronic renal impairment, renal vein thrombosis, sepsis, etc. Hemorrhagic areas may appear hyperechoic/dense. Striated nephrogram (alternating bands of high and low attenuation corresponding to differential enhancement of infected and normal regions) may be seen in the excretory phase with persistent enhancement on delayed scans due to stasis of contrast through the tubules.

Differential Diagnosis

■ *Renal Infarct*: Wedge-shaped area that spares the cortex, giving a rim sign.

■ Renal abscess

- Cystic renal lesions

Laboratory parameters such as leukocytosis, high ESR, and CRP help differentiate.

Management

- Antibiotics (empiric initially followed by antibiotics according to urine culture report) and symptomatic treatment
- Percutaneous nephrostomy

Case 79 Pyonephrosis

A 42-year-old patient with fever, flank pain, and dysuria (Figure 3.14).

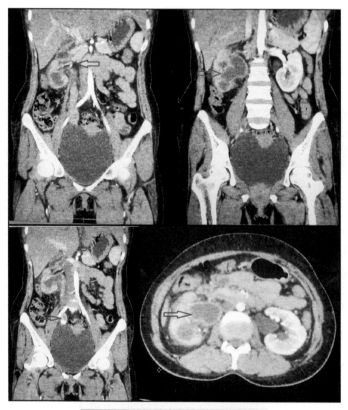

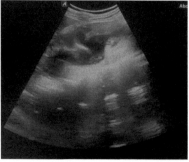

Figure 3.14   (a) CECT abdomen shows distal right ureteric calculus with moderate upstream dilatation of PCS, renal pelvic wall thickening and enhancement, cortical thinning, and perirenal and periureteric fat stranding. Non-excretion of contrast in the excretory phase, even after 24 hours, suggests a non-functioning kidney. (b) Sonography of the right kidney shows dependent echogenic debris in the dilated calyceal system.

Discussion

Pyonephrosis is purulent debris in a dilated renal PCS, along with the destruction of renal parenchyma, with partial or complete loss of renal function. The risk factors include the ascending migration of bacteria through the urethra, bladder, ureter, and kidneys, especially in patients with immunosuppression, renal failure, drainage devices, etc. Patients may present with fever, flank pain, and characteristic imaging findings. Sonography shows calculi, moving internal echoes/urine-debris levels//gas with reverberation artifacts within the obstructed and dilated PCS. CT reveals a thickened pelvic wall (> 2 mm), parenchymal and perinephric fat stranding/inflammatory changes, calculi, and dilated obstructed PCS with purulent debris/gas-fluid/fluid-fluid levels with high HU values. CT urography depicts an indistinct renal outline in a non-functioning kidney.

Differential Diagnosis

The lesion should be differentiated by etiology—pyogenic, tubercular, or fungal causes.

Management

Percutaneous nephrostomy tube drainage
Surgery, if indicated.

Case 80 Ureterosciatic Hernia (Curlicue Ureter)

A 62-year-old female presented with lower abdominal pain (Figure 3.15).

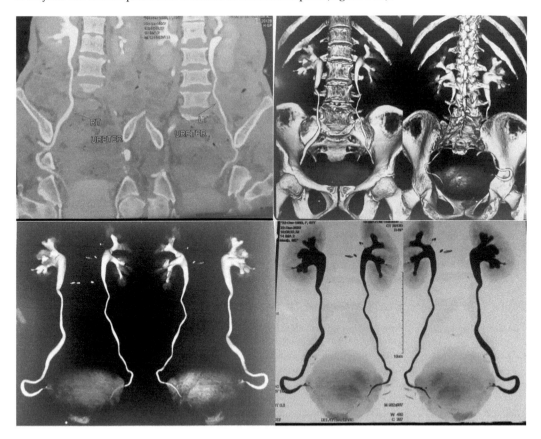

Figure 3.15 CT IVU images in supine and prone positions depict an abnormal curled course of bilateral lower ureters. Reconstructed image shows herniation of the ureter through the greater sciatic notch bilaterally—"Curlicue" ureter.

Discussion

Uretero-sciatic (Lindblom) hernias are extremely rare variants where ureters herniate in the supra-piriformis compartment of the greater sciatic foramen (posterior pelvic wall) depicted as a curled and tortuous ureter with the bend of the herniated ureter passing laterally to the medial wall of the bony pelvis on the urogram. The patients may be asymptomatic or may present with flank pain due to ureteral obstruction. Risk factors include hip joint-related piriformis muscle atrophy, defective pelvic fascia, adhesions, neuromuscular disorders, etc.

Management

Asymptomatic patients: Observation
Symptomatic patients with severe ureteral obstruction: Stenting or surgery.

Case 81 Renal Trauma

A 25-year-old male with a stab injury (Figure 3.16).

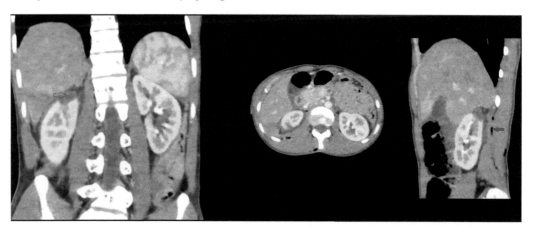

Figure 3.16 CECT abdomen depicts linear laceration (open arrow), small subcapsular hematoma (arrowhead), and mild hemoperitoneum (star). Multiple coarse air foci in the right paraspinal muscle with skin irregularities (solid arrow).

Discussion

Kidneys remain protected and cushioned owing to their retroperitoneal location, though trauma is noted after blunt and penetrating injuries. Patients may present with hematuria, hypotension, fractured ribs, and lumbar vertebrae. Parenchymal lacerations and de-vascularized segments are best seen in the early nephrographic phase.

Table 3.7 depicts the radiological pattern of different types of injuries.

Table 3.7: Radiological Pattern of Different Types of Injuries.

Contusion	Ill-defined hypodense area; enhancement is less on the nephrographic phase but persists on delayed enhancement
Infarcts	Wedge-shaped hypodense non-enhancing region
Subcapsular hematoma	Crescentic/biconvex blood collection, flattens the renal contour
Perinephric hematoma	Blood collection between the renal parenchyma and Gerota's fascia without flattening the renal contour
Lacerations	Irregular, linear, non-enhancing hypodense regions of parenchymal discontinuity
Shattered kidney	Multiple lacerations with fragmented parenchyma, collecting duct injuries, and devascularized vascular pedicle
Pseudoaneurysm	Localized, well-circumscribed lesion that shows intense arterial enhancement similar to blood pool phase
Active arterial extravasation	An ill-defined, localized area of contrast leak is hyperdense than the blood pool phase and expands on the delayed scan
Urinary extravasation	a/w PCS injury and best seen in 3–5 minutes delayed scan

Management

Depends on hemodynamic stability

■ *Grade 1–4 Injuries*: Conservative and percutaneous drainage

■ *Severe*: Surgical repair

Case 82 Shattered Kidney

A 30-year-old male with blunt abdominal trauma and hematuria (Figure 3.17).
  Discussion (Last case)

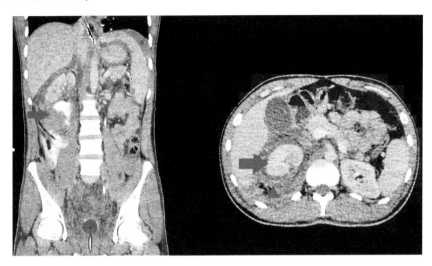

Figure 3.17 CECT abdomen depicts laceration at right upper pole with disrupted mid and lower pole of kidney (arrow) with fragments displaced inferiorly by a large hyperattenuating perinephric collection (arrowhead) with contrast extravasation, thickened fascias, and adjacent fat stranding due to PUJ disruption. Moderate hemoperitoneum (star).

Case 83 Renal Artery Stenosis with Renal Parenchymal Disease

A 48-year-old patient with hypertension (Figure 3.18).

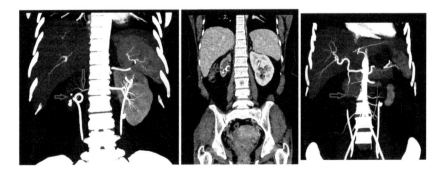

Figure 3.18 CTU reveals a relatively attenuated caliber of the right renal artery with delayed nephrogram in the right kidney s/o RAS. No flow-limiting thrombus is noted. Asymmetric nephrogram with small contracted right kidney showing delayed contrast uptake, reduced renal cortical thickness, and partial loss of cortico-medullary differentiation s/o RPD. Normal nephrogram and prompt excretion of contrast in left kidney. Left upper ureteric calculus and bilateral renal calculi. No hydronephrosis in either kidney or collecting system. DJ stents in situ in bilateral collecting systems.

Discussion

Renal artery stenosis (RAS) is a major cause of secondary hypertension, the most common etiology being atherosclerosis (ostial/proximal narrowing of the renal artery, common in the older age groups)

and the second most common cause being fibromuscular dysplasia (FMD, common in young females). The arterial narrowing results in ischemia and reduced renal function. Patients present with resistant or malignant hypertension with altered renal function even after antihypertensive therapy. The other essential signs include epigastric bruit and recurrent flash pulmonary edema.

Imaging shows asymmetric renal atrophy with a difference of > 1.5 cm between the two kidneys. CDUS shows peak systolic velocity (PSV) >180 cm/s, renal artery/aorta velocity ratio (RAR) >3.5, parvus tardus (slow) flow. On angiography, vessel plaque at the origin of the renal artery results in stenosis due to atherosclerosis. FMD causes medial fibroplasia at the distal two-thirds of the renal vessel with the appearance of a string of beads.

Renal transplant patients should be observed for worsening renal function and refractory hypertension due to RAS. The other causes of RAS include vasculitis, Takayasu's arteritis, coarctation of the abdominal aorta, and aortic dissection.

Differential Diagnosis

- Primary hypertension in adults due to other causes
- Hypertension in children may occur due to neurofibromatosis, William's syndrome, and middle aortic syndrome
- Renal parenchymal disease due to other causes

Management

- Medical management
- Stent placement
- Angioplasty
- Surgical revascularization in a few cases

Case 84 Hypoplastic Right Kidney

A 30-year-old male incidentally noted a small kidney on sonography and CECT for further evaluation (Figure 3.19).

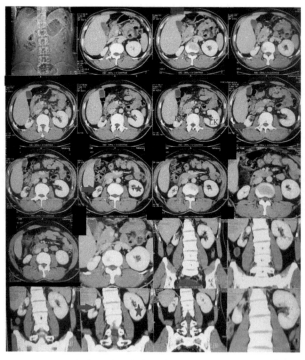

Figure 3.19   CECT abdomen depicts a hypoplastic right kidney.

Discussion

Hypoplastic/small-sized kidney refers to a uni/bilateral decrease in renal mass/volume. Unilateral hypoplastic kidney usually functions normally and a/w compensatory contralateral hypertrophy. Hypoplastic kidneys have normal renal parenchyma with smaller calyces, papillae, etc., and secrete less quantity of urine though with normal constituents. There can be global or focal renal hypoplasia. On imaging, the hypoplastic kidney is small in size with normal contours, echogenicity, and CMD but is vulnerable to infections and calculi formation.

Differential Diagnosis

- Congenital hypoplasia

- Reflux nephropathy

- Renovascular ischemia

- Chronic pyelonephritis (irregular contour and scarring)

- Partial nephrectomy

Management

- Regular follow-up assessments

- Endoscopic interventions/surgery depending on the complications

Case 85 Ruptured Angiomyolipoma

A 39-year-old female presented to the emergency department with acute onset, progressively worsening left-sided abdominal pain after exercise. She was hypotensive and diaphoretic (Figure 3.20).

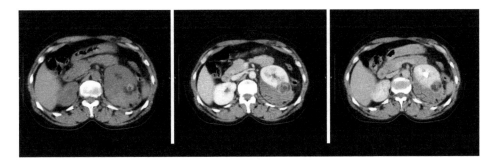

Figure 3.20 CT depicts heterogeneous (star), mixed attenuation (macroscopic fat-arrow) in the lower pole of the left kidney with retroperitoneal, perirenal hematoma (open arrow) causing anterior displacement of the left kidney.

Discussion

Angiomyolipoma (AML) is the most frequent mesenchymal tumor, a benign neoplasm with perivascular epithelioid differentiation (PEComa) that constitutes fat, smooth muscle, and blood vessels. It has a propensity to increase in size during pregnancy due to its hormone-sensitive nature. The lack of elastic membrane and hypervascular nature with tortuous blood vessels in this tumor makes it prone to pseudoaneurysm formation and rupture, causing retroperitoneal bleeding, especially if the size is more than 4 cm. It may rupture even with trivial trauma, mild exercise, or abdominal palpation. Patients present with Lenk's triad of flank mass, acute abdominal pain, and hypovolemic shock. Sonography depicts high echogenicity due to fat, which CT corroborates with a negative HU value. Doppler may show color flow with to and fro pattern if the lesion is a/w pseudoaneurysm.

Differential Diagnosis

1. Young female/pregnant presenting to emergency with hypotensive shock makes ruptured ectopic pregnancy a vital differential.

2. AVM rupture

3. Hemorrhagic ovarian torsion/rupture

Management

Asymptomatic AMLs<4 cm: Observation
Bleeding AMLs/size>4 cm: Renal artery embolization or surgery

Case 86 Multilocular Cystic Nephroma (MLCN)

A 42-year-old male patient presented with abdominal pain and a palpable mass (Figure 3.21).

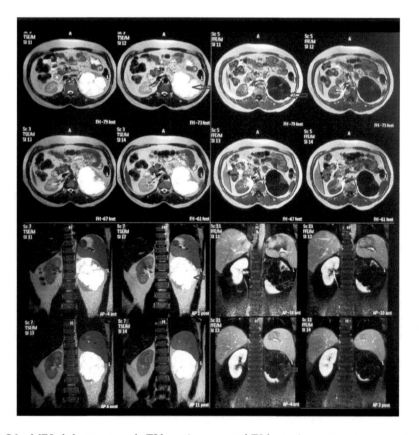

Figure 3.21 MRI abdomen reveals TI hypointense and T2 hyperintense noncommunicating cystic lesions in the left kidney.

Discussion

Multilocular cystic nephroma (MLCN), a slow-growing, unilateral, benign mixed mesenchymal and epithelial renal neoplasm with premalignant potential, may present with abdominal pain, palpable mass, or remain asymptomatic and discovered incidentally during imaging.

A plain X-ray shows a large abdominal lesion displacing the bowel loops. Sonography reveals a multilocular, anechoic cystic mass with irregular septations of varying thickness and vascularity. The cysts do not communicate with the renal pelvis and may contain low-level echoes. CT depicts a well-defined, non-enhancing cystic lesion with enhancing septations. The claw sign or beak shape corroborates the renal origin of the lesion. Occasionally, the lesion may herniate into the renal pelvis, leading to obstructive dilatation of calyces. MRI shows a fluid-intensity cystic mass with septal enhancement.

Differential Diagnosis

Cystic RCC
Unilateral PCKD

Management

Radical/partial nephrectomy

Case 87 Renal Cell Carcinoma

A 56-years-old male with hematuria and flank pain (Figure 3.22).

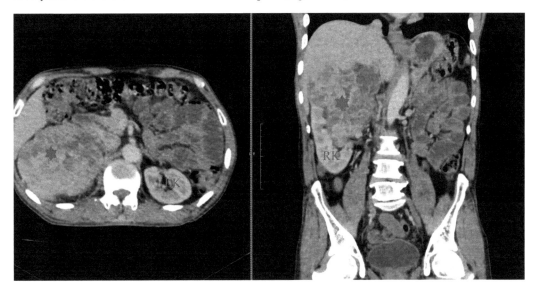

Figure 3.22 CECT abdomen depicts a well-defined, lobulated, partially exophytic heterogeneously enhancing solid lesion in the upper and mid pole of the kidney.

Discussion

RCC, hypernephroma, is the commonest primary renal malignancy, adenocarcinoma in nature, frequent in elderly males who usually present with hematuria, palpable mass, and flank pain; the common risk factors being smoking, hypertension, obesity, and history of dialysis/renal transplant. RCC is a/w hereditary syndromes (Von Hippel Lindau and Birt-Hogg-Dube) and paraneoplastic syndromes (polycythemia, hypercalcemia, Stauffer syndrome, etc).

Histopathological subtypes of RCC (Table 3.8).

Table 3.8: Histopathological Subtypes of RCC

Clear cell carcinoma (cortex)	75%	Hypervascular, expansile tumor; Large cells with clear cytoplasm
Papillary	15%	Hypovascular (simulates cysts), multifocal, bilateral, a/w chronic hemodialysis
Chromophobe	4%	Central scar (simulates oncocytoma); best prognosis
Bellini duct (collecting duct)	<1%	Worst prognosis: young patients
Medullary carcinoma	rare	a/w sickle cell disease/trait

On imaging, the lesions are heterogeneous with solid-cystic bean type (maintains the reniform contour) or ball type (expansile mass distorting the renal shape). Sonography is better at differentiating cystic lesions and septations. NCCT scans show areas of calcification and necrosis. CECT better delineates the extensions into the perinephric fat, renal vein, IVC, adjacent muscles, and organs. Hematogenous metastasis is common in the lungs and bone. The nephrogenic phase of CT urography is sensitive in discerning contrast enhancement. The lesion is T1 hypointense T2 hyperintense and shows restricted diffusion.

Differential Diagnosis

- Renal AML contains macroscopic fat.

- Renal lymphoma may present as an infiltrative type lesion or multiple less-enhancing lesions in bilaterally enlarged kidneys.

- TCC (urothelial carcinoma) involves the renal collecting system.

- Multilocular cystic nephroma

- Complex renal cyst

- Renal abscess

- Metastasis

Management

- Partial nephrectomy

- Radiofrequency/cryo/chemical ablation

Case 88 Infiltrating Bladder Carcinoma

A 56-year-old patient with hematuria (Figure 3.23).

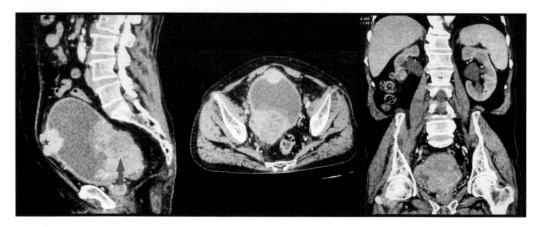

Figure 3.23 CECT abdomen depicts an ill-defined polypoidal infiltrative intraluminal heterogeneously enhancing mass (solid arrow) lesion arising from the right postero-lateral wall infiltrating (arrowhead) prostate and right seminal vesicle with encasement of right vesicoureteric junction causing mild upstream right hydroureteronephrosis (open arrow) and mild perivesical fat stranding. Another relatively well-defined heterogeneously enhancing mass (star) lesion in the anterior wall of the urinary bladder with focal infiltration of the right rectus abdominis muscle. Left kidney is normal with mild left hydroureteronephrosis.

Discussion

TCCs, urothelial carcinomas, are frequent in elderly males and smokers, with exposure to amines, polycyclic hydrocarbons, cyclophosphamide, and chronic infection. More than two-thirds are superficial (intact detrusor with good prognosis), and the rest are invasive (invades lamina propria with poor prognosis). Tumors can be polypoidal or sessile, are frequently multifocal, and prone to recurrence. Adjacent structures such as perivesical fat and other pelvic organs may be invaded along with distant metastasis to lymph nodes (common iliac and para-aortic nodes), lungs, bones, and liver. The other rare varieties are squamous cell, small cell, and adenocarcinoma. Imaging of TCC depicts focal/generalized asymmetric thickening of the bladder wall or polypoidal masses protruding into the bladder lumen or invading the adjacent tissues, depending on the tumor staging. Patients with associated BPH should be evaluated carefully. Sonography shows echogenic thickening, which has to be differentiated from the hematoma, that changes its position with variation in the patient's position compared to malignancy. CT/MRI better delineates the adjacent spread, and the delayed phase (urography) is better for identifying tumor enhancement. CT scan, especially CTU (urography), is the most commonly used imaging modality to assess regional, nodal, and distant metastatic spread. The lesion is T1 isointense, T2 hyperintense, and shows enhancement. Multiparametric MRI is better for evaluating the staging of bladder cancer.

Vesical Imaging-Reporting and Data System (VI-RADS) is a standardized format to stage bladder cancer with MRI using T2WI, DWI, and CE-MRI.

- *VI-RADS 1 & 2*: No tumor infiltration with intact muscularis propria
- *VI-RADS 3*: Indeterminate for muscle invasion
- *VI-RADS 4 & 5*: Tumor infiltration and extension beyond the bladder wall

Pitfalls

To avoid the false-positive diagnosis of bladder cancer and over-staging on MRI:

- The bladder should be distended optimally.
- MRI should be done before or at least 2 weeks after cystoscopic procedures or intravesical treatment.
- MRI should be done at least 2 days after catheter removal or in any instrumentation to avoid artifacts from air in the bladder lumen.

Differential Diagnosis

- Benign prostatic hypertrophy
- Carcinoma prostate
- Metastasis
- Bladder hematoma

Management

- The cystoscopic biopsy is diagnostic.
- Superficial tumors have a good prognosis and can be managed by TURBT (Transurethral Resection of Bladder Tumor) +/– intravesical chemotherapy.
- Invasive tumors with poorer prognoses require radical cystectomy, chemotherapy, and external beam radiotherapy.

Case 89 Hutch Diverticula with TCC

A 45-year-old male with painless hematuria (Figure 3.24).

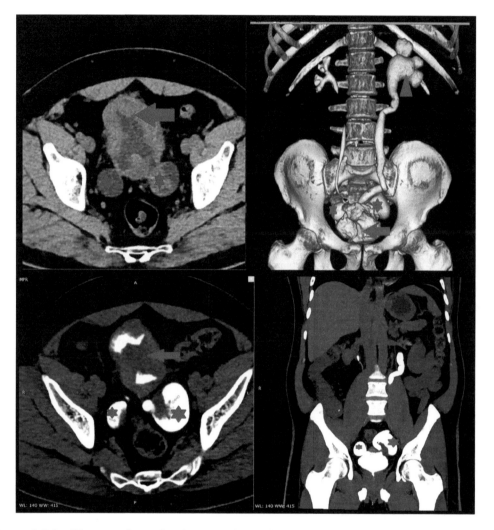

Figure 3.24 CT urography with volume rendering depicts multifocal enhancing lesions (arrow) along the bladder lumen with the extension of malignancy to bilateral Hutch diverticula (star) and left VUJ with mildly dilated ureter and extrarenal pelvis (arrowhead).

Discussion

Tumors are commonly a/w bladder diverticula owing to urinary stasis. Hutch diverticulae are congenital due to defective normal muscle around the ureteric orifice, resulting in the herniation of the bladder mucosa through the detrusor muscle. They are frequent in males, usually asymptomatic, but may present with repeated infections due to calculi formation or urinary retention. Sonography depicts anechoic outpouchings posterolaterally at the trigone base and is better delineated with CT urography. TCC is discussed in the last case.

Differential Diagnosis

Trabeculated bladder due to bladder outlet obstruction.

Management

Prophylactic surgery is advisable due to the high risk of malignancy.

PEDIATRIC

Case 90 Horseshoe Kidney

A 9-year-old boy with an incidental finding on sonography (Figure 3.25).

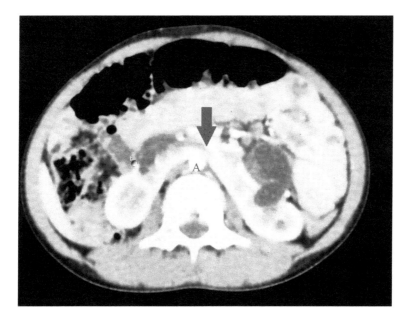

Figure 3.25 CECT abdomen reveals fusion of the renal parenchyma, with two distinct kidneys on each side of the midline (solid arrow) with the aorta (A) posteriorly.

Discussion

Horseshoe kidney is the most prevalent congenital anomaly formed by the fusion of two separate, functional kidneys, one on either side of the midline, mainly at the lower poles. The isthmus of functioning renal parenchyma or fibrous tissue connects them. Normal ascent of kidneys is interrupted by the inferior mesenteric artery, which results in a lower abdominal location and abnormal rotation, especially at the lower poles. The pelvis and ureters are anterior, ventrally crossing the isthmus. Due to its location and poor drainage, the horseshoe kidney is susceptible to trauma and complications such as hydronephrosis due to PUJ obstruction, renal calculi, infection, and an increased risk for malignancies. Poor visualization of the bilateral lower poles on a USG ought to caution the sonographer to seek aberrant tissue that might be the isthmus, which could be mistaken for preaortic mass/lymph node or underestimated renal length. CT/MRI aids in delineating the structural and functional anatomy and early identification of complications.

Differential Diagnosis

■ Crossed fused ectopia
■ Malrotated kidney

Management

Patients with horseshoe kidneys typically have an expected lifespan and don't need any intervention. It's critical to acknowledge their existence before undergoing any surgical/interventional procedures for the abdomen.

Case 91 Crossed Fused Ectopia

A 15-year-old child with an incidental finding on sonography (Figure 3.26).

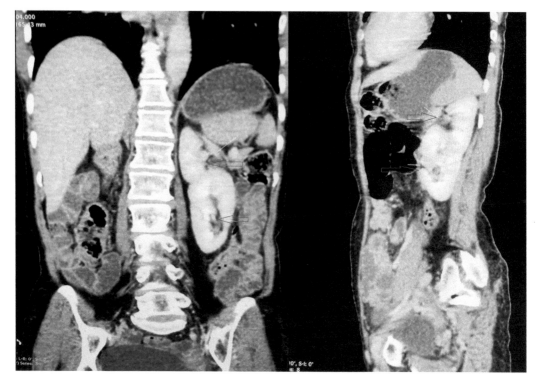

Figure 3.26 CECT abdomen depicts an empty right renal fossa. The right kidney is noted in the left lumbar region, fusing its upper pole with the left kidney's lower pole. Both hilums are malrotated, facing anterolaterally.

Discussion

A normal kidney reaches the L2 level around the fourth to eighth weeks of gestation. Crossed fused renal ectopia is an anomaly due to abnormal renal ascent (due to an anomalous umbilical artery) during embryogenesis, resulting in ipsilateral fused kidneys.

Sonography depicts an absent renal fossa on one side with anterior/posterior notches due to the altered orientation of PCSs of two fused kidneys. It may reveal complications due to calyceal distortion, hydronephrosis, calculi, and vascular supply.

The parenchymal fused band is better depicted on CT, and anomalous vascular supply is better depicted on CT angiogram. The ectopic kidney can fuse superior or inferior to the normal kidney in a sigmoid (S) or L or disc shape.

Management

No intervention is required.

Case 92 Multicystic Dysplastic Kidney

A 7-month-old female with urinary tract infection (Figure 3.27).

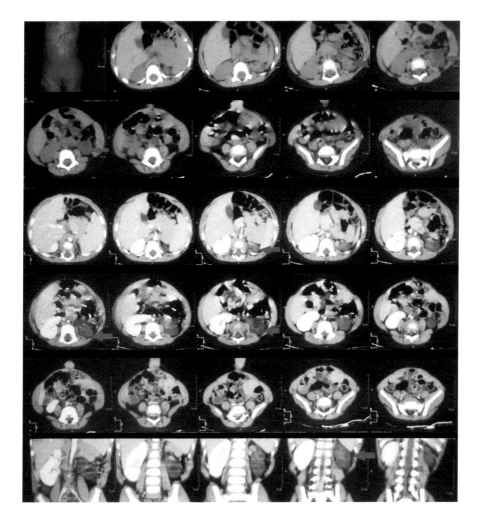

Figure 3.27 CECT abdomen depicting multiple cystic lesions in a non-functioning left kidney.

Discussion

MCDK, severe renal dysplasia, occurs due to defective synchronization between ureteric bud and metanephric blastema, resulting in a non-functioning kidney. Unilateral anomaly has a better prognosis, though the contralateral kidney may have complications such as VUR, etc., compared to bilateral disease, which is almost always fatal.

Two varieties

1. *Pelvi-Infundibular Type*: Replacement of normal renal parenchyma with multiple noncommunicating cysts of varying sizes, echogenic cortex, and ureteric atresia.

2. *Hydronephrotic Type*: dominant cyst in the renal pelvis.

Imaging reveals noncommunicating cysts of varying sizes with echogenic, thinned-out cortex and poor CMD. The kidney may be complicated by infection or hypertension.

Differential Diagnosis

- Hydronephrosis
- Cystic renal tumor
- Unilateral ADPCKD
- PUJ obstruction

Management

- Conservative approach with follow-up serial sonography and monitoring for hypertension
- Surgery in complicated cases

Case 93 Posterior Urethral Valve with VUR

A male child with recurrent urinary tract infections (Figure 3.28).

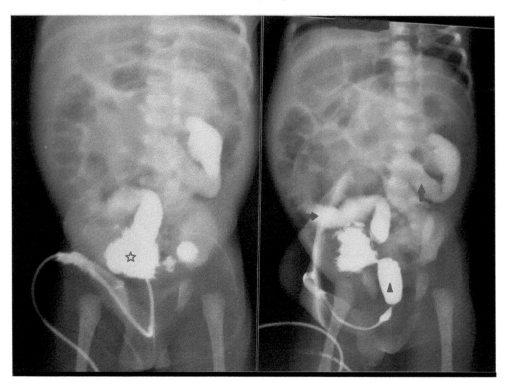

Figure 3.28 VCUG shows dilated posterior urethra (arrowhead) with hypertrophied and trabeculated bladder (star) and bilateral high-grade vesicoureteral reflux (arrows).

Discussion

Posterior urethral valve is the most common cause of bladder outlet obstruction in males. The child presents with difficulty in urination and abnormal growth. Antenatal sonography reveals oligohydramnios, a 'key-hole' sign due to dilated posterior urethra and hypertrophied distended bladder. Pulmonary hypoplasia is noted in severe cases. Postnatal sonography shows a dilated posterior urethra, thickened trabeculated bladder wall, bilateral hydroureteronephrosis, and urinoma/ascites in case of rupture. Hyperechoic kidneys with loss of corticomedullary differentiation suggest renal damage. VCUG, the gold standard modality, shows dilated and elongated posterior urethra, linear radiolucent valve, trabeculated bladder, hydroureteronephrosis, and vesicoureteral reflux.

Reflux is graded depending on the level of reflux (Table 3.9).

Table 3.9: Grading of Reflux in VUR

Grade I	Reflux confined to ureters
Grade II	Reflux involving the renal pelvis
Grade III	Reflux with mild hydroureteronephrosis
Grade IV	Reflux with moderate hydroureteronephrosis with blunted fornices and preserved papillary impressions
Grade V	Reflux with severe tortuous hydroureteronephrosis with loss of fornices and papillary impressions

Management

- Vesicoamniotic shunting antenatally
- Transurethral valve ablation

Case 94 Anterior Urethral Valve

One-year-old male strains during passing urine (Figure 3.29).

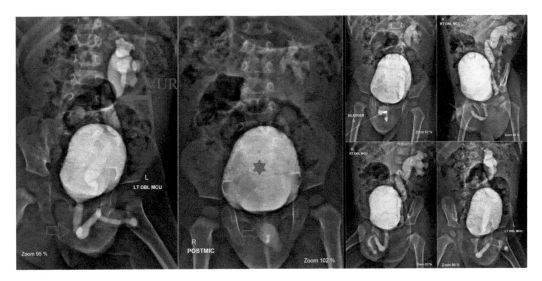

Figure 3.29 VCUG depicts dilated urethra up to mid penile region with linear filling defect and normal rest of the urethra. High-grade vesicoureteric reflux with dilated ureter and pelvis on the left side during micturition (solid arrow). Significant post-void residual contrast in the bladder (star).

Discussion

Congenital anterior urethral valve, posteriorly directed semilunar fold, is a rare cause of infra-vesical lower urinary tract obstruction common in the male urethra (bulbar > penile > penoscrotal junction).

VCUG shows the valve as a linear filling defect, dilated anterior urethra proximal to the valve and distal narrowing, hypertrophied bladder neck, VUR, and urethral diverticulum. Urethroscopy corroborates the diagnosis.

Management

Transurethral valve ablation

Case 95 Supernumerary Kidneys

Rare finding (Figure 3.30).

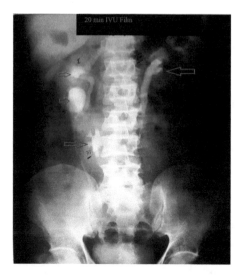

Figure 3.30 IVU film at 20 minutes reveals four kidneys (arrows)—one on the left and three on the right.

Discussion

Supernumerary kidneys are a rare anomaly in which accessory kidneys are small-sized with reduced excretion. Sonography depicts morphological evaluation, and other modalities, such as IVU, CT, MRI, and nuclear scans, may help assess the functional nature of kidneys. These kidneys are not fused and have their own blood supply and capsule with an asymmetric collecting system and variable ureteric drainage. It can have a bifid ureter when the accessory kidney lies caudally or separate ureters when it lies cranial to the normal kidney. Complications such as hydronephrosis, calculi, pyelonephritis, etc, should be considered. Appropriate reporting should include exact number, position, orientation, size, vascular supply, and excretory function.

Differential Diagnosis

Duplex kidney (fused with ipsilateral kidney. May have two PCSs).

Management

Asymptomatic Cases: Regular sonography follow-ups

Case 96 Wilms Tumor

A two-year-old female patient presented with a palpable abdominal mass (Figure 3.31).

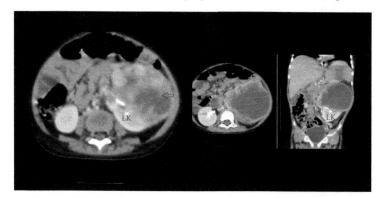

Figure 3.31 CECT abdomen depicts an enlarged left kidney with lobulated, heterogeneously enhancing lesion in the upper and mid pole with renal sinus invasion and displacement of adjacent structures.

Discussion

Wilm's tumor/nephroblastoma, an embryonic renal neoplasm, frequently presents with abdominal mass, hematuria, pain, etc. It is commonly a/w the following syndromes.

- WAGR (Wilms, Aniridia, genitourinary malformations, and mental retardation)

- *Beckwith*: Wiedemann Syndrome (macroglossia, hemihypertrophy, testiculomegaly, etc.)

On imaging, the lesion is well-circumscribed and heterogenous with fluid, fat, and calcifications, showing patchy enhancement. Sonography shows heterogeneously echogenic lesions. CT helps delineate the claw sign, suggesting the renal origin apart from the extent of local and distant spread. The lesion is isointense on T1 and hyperintense on T2. It may metastasize to lymph nodes, contralateral kidney, lung, liver, bones, etc.

Differential Diagnosis

- *Mesoblastic Nephroma*: Usually noted in the neonate.

- Neuroblastoma (Table 3.10)

- *Rhabdoid Tumor*: a/w brain tumors

- Cystic nephroma (challenging to differentiate from cystic Wilm's tumor) (Table 3.10)

Table 3.10: **Nephroblatoma vs Neuroblastoma**

	Nephroblastoma (Wilm's)	Neuroblastoma
Age	< 5 years	< 2 years
Origin	Renal	Adrenal (primordial neural crest cells)
Effect on the collecting system	Distorts; claw sign shows the intrarenal origin	Extrinsic mass effect
Renal veins & IVC/ vasculature	Invasion	Encasement lifts the aorta anteriorly, away from the spine
Calcifications	Less frequent	More frequent
Margins	Well-circumscribed	Poorly marginated
Common site for metastasis	Lungs	Bones

Management

Nephrectomy and chemotherapy

SUGGESTED READINGS

Drake, R. L., & Vogl, A. W. (2020). *Gray's Atlas of Anatomy E-Book*. Elsevier Health Sciences.

Houat, A. P., Guimarães, C. T. S., Takahashi, M. S., Rodi, G. P., Gasparetto, T. P. D., Blasbalg, R., & Velloni, F. G. Congenital anomalies of the upper urinary tract: A comprehensive review. *RadioGraphics* 2021;41:2:462–486.

Lee, J. K. T. (2006). *Computed Body Tomography with MRI Correlation*. Lippincott Williams & Wilkins.

Lumley, J. S., & Craven, J. L. (2018). *Bailey & Love's Essential Clinical Anatomy*. CRC Press.

Saba, L., & Suri, J. S. (2022). *Multi-Detector CT Imaging Handbook, Two Volume Set*. CRC Press.

4 Adrenal Glands

INTRODUCTION

Embryology

The adrenal cortex arises from the suprarenal ridge, formed by the celomic epithelium (mesoderm) growth on each side of the primitive gut's root of the dorsal mesentery. The ridge runs from the sixth to the twelfth thoracic segments. The cortical cells initially have acidophilic cytoplasm, and later, basophilic cytoplasmic cells cover the fetal cortex, which divides into three cell zones.

The medulla is formed from the neuro-ectoderm of the ventral portion of the primordial spinal ganglia, which is produced from neural crest cells. The cells shift ventrally, enter the suprarenal ridge, and remain in the medulla as chromaffin cells (Figure 4.1).

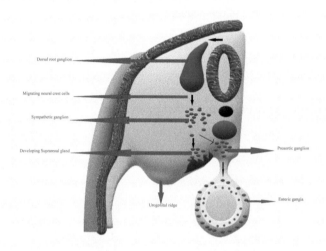

Figure 4.1 Embryology of adrenal glands.

Anatomy

Adrenal glands are the paired, retroperitoneal, endocrine glands in the posterior abdominal wall on each side of the vertebral column lying supero-anteromedially to the kidneys. Each gland has an outer cortex and inner medulla, which differ structurally, functionally, and developmentally.

Mesoderm: outer cortex (zona glomerulosa-mineralocorticoids, zona fasciculata-glucocorticoids, and zona reticularis-sex steroids)

Neural crest—inner medulla (catecholamines)

Measurements

Height—50 mm, breadth—30 mm, thickness—10 mm, and weigh approximately 5 g. Fetal adrenal glands are proportionately larger (about one-third of the size of the kidney) compared to the adult gland, which forms one-thirteenth of the kidney's size. The right suprarenal gland is pyramidal, the left suprarenal gland is semilunar, and concavity is directed laterally.

Arterial Supply

Suprarenal arteries

- *Superior*: Branch of the inferior phrenic artery

- *Middle*: Abdominal aorta

- *Inferior*: Renal arteries

Venous Drainage

- *Right Suprarenal Vein*: IVC

- *Left Suprarenal Vein*: Left renal/inferior phrenic vein

- **Lymphatics**

- Para-aortic nodes

- **Innervation**

- Splanchnic nerves from aortic and renal plexus

- **Technical pitfalls**

- *Size of ROI*: Should cover two-thirds of the lesion.

- Smaller ROI (to determine microscopic fat) may give imprecise results due to intralesional heterogeneity.

- Exclude the peripheral area of the nodule to avoid partial volume average artifact from the retroperitoneal fat.

- Tube voltage selection affects density measurements of soft tissues (usually 120 kVp for adrenal glands). Automated tube voltage may lead to variable tube voltage and erroneous density measurements.

- The timing of contrast-enhanced imaging is critical.

Case 97 Adrenal Adenoma

A 44-year-old patient with an incidental finding (Figure 4.2).

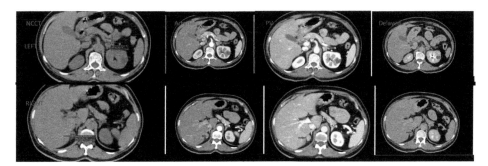

Figure 4.2   CT abdomen depicts well-defined ovoid hypodense lesions (average –10–65 HU) and rapid contrast washout in the lateral limb of the right adrenal and body of the left adrenal gland. AW is 77% and 74% in the right and left, respectively. RW is 57% and 55% in right and left lesions.

Discussion

Adenomas are the most frequent adrenal tumors arising from the adrenal cortex and are commonly seen as incidentalomas (Figure 4.2). Benign, non-functioning adenomas with normal hormonal levels are frequently compared to functional adenomas a/w endocrine disorders. Adenomas are usually < 3–4 cm, homogeneous, well-circumscribed, and consist of clear cells with intracytoplasmic fat.

CT washout is important in evaluating adrenal adenomas. CSI is pivotal in discerning intralesion fat. DECT allows virtual non-contrast (VNC) and iodine density measurements and helps characterize adrenal lesions.

Absolute washout (AW) = (CE-DE/CE-NC) * 100
Relative washout (RW) = (CE-DE/CE) * 100
NC (HU): Non-contrast
CE (HU): Contrast enhancement at 60–70 seconds
DE (HU): Delayed enhancement at 15 minutes
Adenomas
AW > 60%
RW > 40%

Differential Diagnosis

Discussed in Table 4.1.

Table 4.1: Differential Diagnoses of Adrenal Lesions

	Lipid-Rich Adenoma	Lipid-Poor Adenoma	Metastasis	Pheochromocytoma	Cyst	Myelolipoma	Malignancy	Hemorrhage
NECT (HU)	<10	>20	>45	Heterogeneous	0–20	Macroscopic fat	>45 Bulky, irregular	40–60
CECT	Rapid enhancement Rapid washout		Rapid/intense enhancement	Peak enhancement>110 HU	Low-level enhancement		Heterogeneous enhancement Rapid washout	No enhancement
Washout	AW>60% RW>40%	AW>60% RW>40%	Prolonged washout	Slow washout				
CSI (chemical shift MRI)	Signal intensity drop of>20%		No signal loss on out-of-phase imaging			Absent out-of-phase loss of signal intensity		
Additional findings	Low-intermediated signal on T2WI		FDG (PET/CTbetter)	High T2WI (Lightbulb sign) I-MIBG scintigraphy 68Ga-DOTANOC PET/CT	MRI Low T1SI and high T2SI	Isointense to retroperitoneal fat on MRI (high on T1 and T2WI) that disappears on fat-suppression techniques	FDG (PET/CT better) Renal vein and IVC invasion Regional and distant spread DWI restriction	a/w trauma, coagulation disorders, stress, severe illness Periadrenal infiltration/haziness

Differentials for absent out-of-phase signal loss in a nodule + T1 iso intensity relative to retroperitoneal fat

- Myelolipoma
- Hemorrhage
- Proteinaceous fluid within a cyst.

Frequency-encoded fat-suppressed MRI sequences or CT may be of use to help confirm the presence of bulk fat.

Signal Intensity Drop at CSI

- Adenomas
- Lipid-rich metastases (large (> 4 cm), heterogeneous lesion with high T2WI size)

Lesions that Cause CT Washout and Mimic Adenomas

- Metastases from hypervascular tumors such as RCC, HCC (large, heterogeneous, irregular lesion with invasion to other structures)
- Pheochromocytomas (biochemical testing—24-hour urine fractionated metanephrine or catecholamine values, and MIBG scanning). High T2WI with absent intracytoplasmic fat)
- Primary malignancy

Non-Adrenal Lesions Mimicking Adrenal Lesions

- Thickened diaphragmatic crura
- Gastric lesions such as gastric diverticula and exophytic gastric tumors (GISTs)
- Splenic lobulation, accessory splenic tissue, tortuous, and aneurysmal splenic vessels
- Renal lesions (Upper pole) (Claw sign helps to differentiate)
- Pancreatic tail lesions
- Exophytic hepatic lesions
- Retroperitoneal liposarcoma (simulates myelolipoma) (Table 4.1)

Case 98 Adrenal Infarcts

A 65-year-old male with severe backache and hypotension (Figure 4.3).

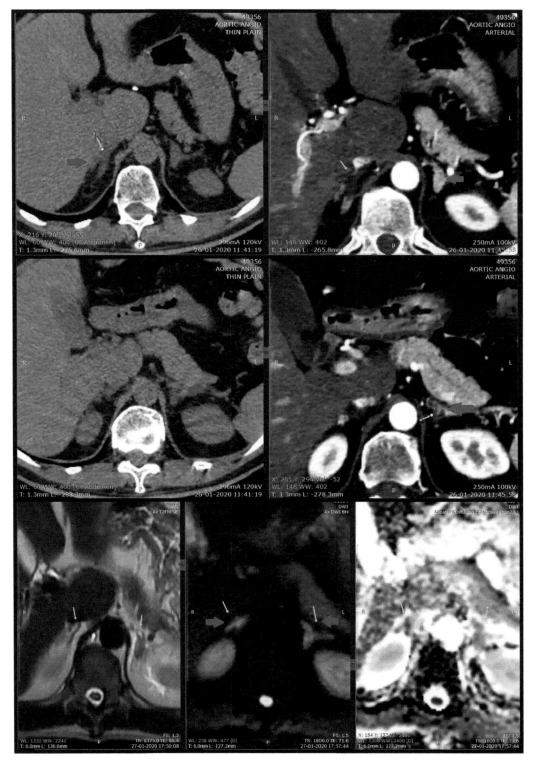

Figure 4.3 CT abdomen reveals hypoattenuating non-enhancing right adrenal gland and mildly enlarged left adrenal with adjacent stranding. T2WI shows hypointense glands with adjacent hyperintense fluid, restricted diffusion on DWI, and corresponding hypointensity on ADC.

Discussion

Adrenal infarct can be uni/bilateral; the various causes include pregnancy, coronavirus, and hypercoagulable state. Waterhouse Friderichsen syndrome constitutes bilateral hemorrhagic adrenal gland infarction due to bilateral adrenal vein thrombosis. Patients may present with severe backache and primary adrenal insufficiency in bilateral cases.

CT imaging depicts hypoattenuating non-enhancing areas in the enlarged adrenals with adjacent fat stranding. T2WI shows hypointense adrenals with adjacent hyperintense edema/inflammatory changes. The diagnosis can be confirmed by restricted diffusion (hyperintensity) on DWI-MRI and corresponding hypointensity on ADC.

Management

Steroid therapy; treatment depends on the etiology

Case 99 Adrenal Hemorrhage

A 45-year-old male with h/o trauma (Figure 4.4).

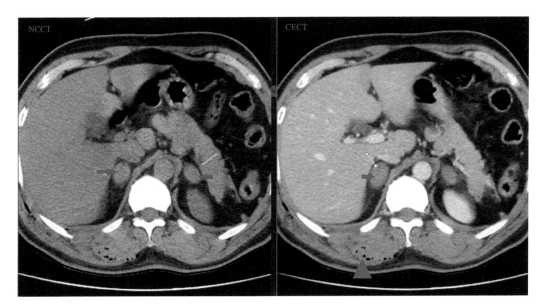

Figure 4.4 CT abdomen depicts non-enhancing bilateral adrenal hemorrhages (arrows) in a patient with subcutaneous emphysema (arrowhead).

Discussion

Adrenal hemorrhage can be traumatic/non-traumatic. Spontaneous bleeding may be noted in hypertensives or patients with any systemic illness, adrenal neoplasm, anticoagulation therapy, or vascular thrombosis. Neonatal adrenal hemorrhage occurs due to traumatic delivery, septicemia, asphyxia, etc.

The hemorrhage is initially heterogeneously hyperechoic/dense on imaging with gradual resorption and reduced echogenicity/density. Hemorrhage is avascular on CDUS and non-enhancing on CECT. Chronic hemorrhage may calcify or liquefy as pseudocysts. MRI characterizes the hemorrhage as acute, subacute, or chronic by different signal intensities on T1- and T2WI.

Differential Diagnosis

Old TB/histoplasmosis. It has to be differentiated from other adrenal lesions depending on the stage of hematoma.

Management

Conservative management with follow-up imaging and close monitoring

Case 100 Adrenal Metastases

Case: A 58-year-old female presented for further evaluation with incidental adrenal and liver lesions on sonography (Figure 4.5).

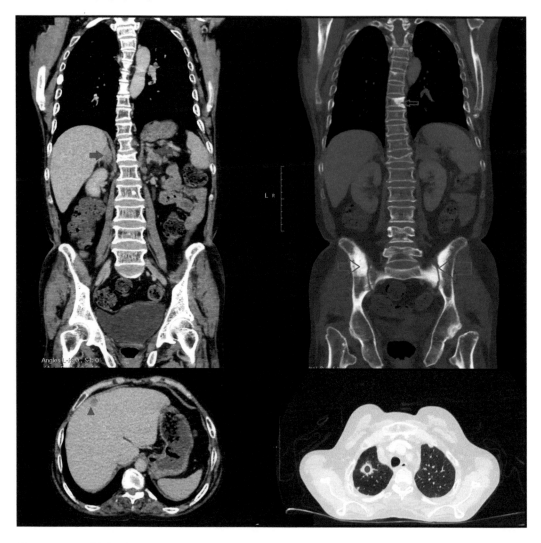

Figure 4.5 CECT abdomen depicts homogeneously enhancing bilateral adrenal lesions (solid arrows), sclerotic bony metastasis (open arrow) in the lung window, focal liver lesion (arrowhead), and primary lung malignancy (circle) in the lung window. FDG-avid lesions with increased uptake and a lung biopsy of the lesion confirmed the findings.

Discussion

The adrenal glands are a common site for metastatic disease, especially in lung cancer. It is frequently solitary, asymptomatic, and found incidentally. Bilateral adrenal metastases occur as a result of the underlying malignancy's systemic dissemination. When incidental adrenal lesions are discovered, especially when bony metastases accompany them, it is imperative to examine the lungs; conversely, it is crucial to monitor the adrenals when checking for lung malignancy in the chest.

When two pathologically distinct tumors, such as adrenal adenoma and metastasis, coexist in the adrenal gland, it is termed an adrenal collision tumor.

Differentials

Discussed in Table 4.1.

Management

Symptomatic relief

Case 101 Extra-adrenal Pheochromocytoma

A 35-year-old female with hypertensive crisis (Figure 4.6).

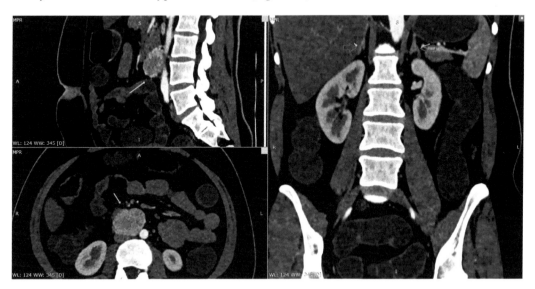

Figure 4.6 CECT abdomen depicts normal bilateral adrenal glands (arrows) and avidly enhancing retroperitoneal (star) pheochromocytoma.

Discussion

Although uncommonly encountered, pheochromocytomas, benign neuroendocrine tumors originating from the adrenal medullary chromaffin cells, are an important cause of uncontrolled secondary hypertension in adults.

A rule of 10 has been ascribed to the epidemiological and morphological spectrum associated with this usually benign tumor.

~10% are extra-adrenal (origin from embryonic neural crest cells and have poor prognosis)

~10% are bilateral

~10% are malignant

~10% are found in children

~10% are not associated with hypertension

~10% contain calcification

Paragangliomas constitute chromaffin cells and extend from the cervical region to the pelvis base along the paravertebral and para-aortic axes. The frequent extra-adrenal sites are the organ of Zuckerkandl (retroperitoneal at the origin of the inferior mesenteric artery), bladder wall, mediastinum, carotid, and glomus jugulare bodies.

Syndromes affiliated to this condition include MEN II A & II B, VHL, NF-1, and Carneys triad. The patients commonly present with headaches, sweating, palpitations, hypertension, and visual disturbances.

On imaging, the lesion appears heteroechoic/dense with varying solid and cystic components, with hemorrhagic areas appearing comparatively hyperechoic/dense. CECT shows significant enhancement on arterial/portal phase images with washout on 15-minute delayed images similar to adrenal adenomas, but adenomas are often <120 HU on an arterial or portal venous contrast phase.

MRI shows the lesion as hypointense on T1WI and homogeneously hyperintense "Light bulb" appearance on T2WI with heterogenous enhancement; however, intralesional necrosis and hemorrhage may cause signal alterations. The differentiation between benign and malignant cases is done based on the invasiveness of the lesion.

MIBG scintigraphy helps diagnose the lesions and assess extra-adrenal involvement and recurrence. Biochemical tests such as increased 24-hour urinary/plasma metanephrines/HVA/VMA confirm the diagnosis.

Differential Diagnosis

Retroperitoneal schwannoma—Heterogeneous enhancement is less compared to avid enhancement and necrosis in highly vascular paraganglioma.

For adrenal pheochromocytomas: Discussed in Table 4.1.

Pitfalls

Clinical symptoms such as hypertensive crisis should be kept in mind before diagnosing finally and to differentiate from other lesions, especially hypervascular metastasis.

Management

Surgical resection is curative with pre-operative medical management with alpha-blockers.

SUGGESTED READINGS

Drake, R. L., & Vogl, A. W. (2020). *Gray's Atlas of Anatomy E-Book*. Elsevier Health Sciences.

Lattin, Jr, G. E., Sturgill, E. D., Tujo, C. A., Marko, J., Sanchez-Maldonado, K. W., Craig, W. D. & Lack, E. E. From the radiologic pathology archives: Adrenal tumors and tumor-like conditions in the adult: Radiologic-pathologic correlation. *RadioGraphics* 2014;34:3, 805–829.

Wang, F., Liu, J., Zhang, R., Bai, Y., Li, C., Li, B., Liu, H., & Zhang, T. CT and MRI of adrenal gland pathologies. *Quant Imaging Med Surg*. 2018;8(8):853–875. doi: 10.21037/qims.2018.09.13.

5 Female Pelvic System (Uterus and Ovaries)

EMBRYOLOGY

The ovary, one on each side, develops within the abdominal cavity from a genital ridge on the posterior abdominal wall. The genital ridge is formed by the thickening of coelomic epithelium that covers the medial side of mesonephros. It receives primordial germ cells derived from the wall of the yolk sac. The ovary then descends into the pelvis with the help of gubernaculum (a band of fibromuscular tissue) and processus vaginalis (a process of the peritoneum formed due to its evagination). The gubernaculum extends from the ovary to the junction of the uterus and uterine tube (forming the ovarian ligament in the adult) and then continues in the labium majus (forming the round ligament of the uterus in the adult). The processus vaginalis is obliterated in the adult.

In an indifferent stage, both pairs of ducts—mesonephric (Wolffian) and paramesonephric (Müllerian) ducts—are present in both the male and the female embryo.

Due to the absence of anti-mullerian hormone (AMH) and SRY gene, the mesonephric ducts disappear in the female embryo. The para-mesonephric ducts persist to form the uterus, fallopian tubes, and upper part of the vagina. The paramesonephric duct arises as a longitudinal invagination of the epithelium on the anterolateral surface of the urogenital ridge. Cranially, the duct opens into the future abdominal cavity. Caudally, it first runs lateral to the mesonephric duct, then crosses it ventrally to grow caudomedially, and fuses with the contralateral paramesonephric duct in the midline. A septum separates the two ducts but later fuses, at around 20 weeks, to form the uterine canal. Failure to resorb the septum results in a septate uterus. The unfused cranial ends form the fallopian tubes with the funnel-shaped fimbrial end. The caudal tip of the combined ducts develops into the upper part of the vagina, and the lower portion is derived from the urogenital sinus. The lumen of the vagina remains separated from that of the urogenital sinus by a thin tissue plate, the hymen, which consists of the epithelial lining of the sinus and a thin layer of vaginal cells. It usually develops a small opening during perinatal life. In short, Mullerian (paramesonephric) duct gives rise to the upper half of the vagina, while the urogenital sinus (sinovaginal bulbs) gives rise to the lower part of the vagina. Two sinovaginal bulbs merge to produce the vaginal plate, which subsequently canalizes to form the vaginal lumen.

The mesonephric duct disappears except for a small cranial portion found in the epoophoron and occasionally a small caudal portion (paroophoron) that may be found in the wall of the uterus or vagina. Later in life, it may form Gartner's cyst. After the ducts fuse in the midline, a broad transverse pelvic fold is established, which extends from the lateral sides of the fused paramesonephric ducts toward the wall of the pelvis, is the broad ligament of the uterus. The uterine tube lies in its upper border, and the ovary lies on its posterior surface. The uterus and broad ligaments divide the pelvic cavity into the uterorectal and uterovesical pouch.

Estrogen stimulates the development of the female external genitalia. The genital tubercle elongates slightly and forms the clitoris; urethral folds do not fuse, as in the male, but develop into the labia minora. Genital swellings enlarge and form the labia majora. The urogenital groove is open and forms the vestibule (Figures 5.1 and 5.2).

ANATOMY

The female reproductive system is divided into internal and external genitalia.

The internal genital organs are situated within the pelvis and include the uterus, cervix, vagina, and pair of ovaries and uterine tubes. The external genital organs in the female are collectively called the vulva and consist of the mons pubis, labia majora and minora, clitoris, vaginal vestibule, and a pair of greater vestibular glands. They form the superficial features of the female perineum.

Uterus and Cervix

- The uterus is pear-shaped, flattened anteroposteriorly, and divided into the body and the cervix. Cornu is the point of fusion between the uterine tube and the body.

- The cervix is the lower cylindrical part that projects into the upper part of the vagina through its anterior wall and is divided into the upper supravaginal part and lower vaginal part.

- Two uterine arteries, two ovarian arteries, and corresponding uterine veins.

- Pre- and para-aortic, external and internal iliac, obturator and sacral nodes.

- Sympathetic and parasympathetic fibers.

DOI: 10.1201/9781003452034-5

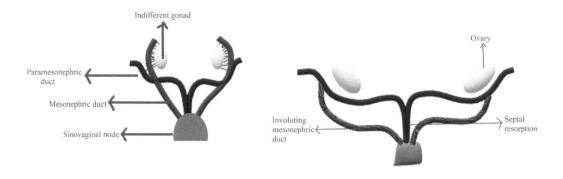

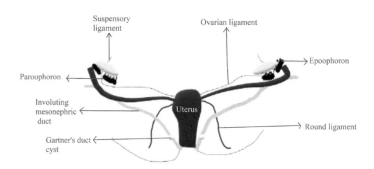

Figure 5.1   Embryology of the female reproductive system.

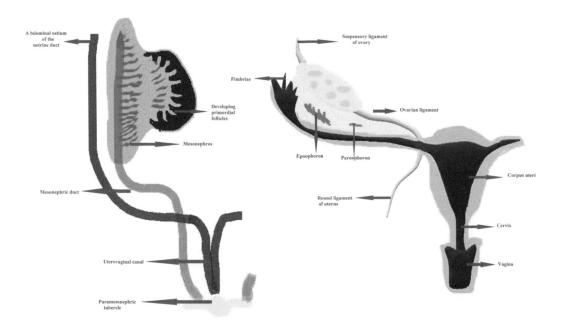

Figure 5.2   Development of female internal genital organs.

Normally, the uterus lies in a position of anteversion and anteflexion.

1. *Anteversion*: The angle of anteversion is a forward angle between the long axis of the cervix and the long axis of the vagina. It measures about 90°.

2. *Anteflexion*: The angle of anteflexion is a forward angle between the long axis of the body of the uterus and the long axis of the cervix at the isthmus. It measures about 120°.

The ligaments of the uterus are classified into two types: false (peritoneal folds) and true (fibromuscular bands). The false ligaments include broad ligaments, rectovaginal fold (posterior ligament), and rectouterine fold (Pouch of Douglas) and do not support the uterus. The true ligaments provide support to the uterus and include the pelvic diaphragm, perineal body, urogenital diaphragm, transverse cervical ligaments (of Mackenrodt), pubocervical ligaments, uterosacral ligaments, and round ligaments of the uterus. The uterine wall consists of three layers from superficial to deep: perimetrium, myometrium, and endometrium.
Normal uterine zonal anatomy. T2WI is ideal.

- *Central Endometrium*: Hyperintense

- Inner myometrium (junctional zone) in continuity with inner fibrous cervical stroma—Hypointense

- Outer myometrium in continuity with outer interstitial cervical stroma—Intermediate SI

Uterine (Fallopian) Tubes

- Pair of ducts that transmit ova from the ovaries to the uterine cavity. From the lateral to medial end, the fallopian tube is divided into four parts:

  - Infundibulum (1 cm long)

  - Ampulla (5 cm long)

  - Isthmus (2.5–3 cm)

  - Intramural (Interstitial) Part (1 cm long)

- Medial two-thirds of the tube is supplied by the uterine artery, and lateral one-third by the ovarian artery.

- Ovarian and uterine veins.

- Internal iliac, pre-aortic, and para-aortic lymph nodes

- Sympathetic and parasympathetic fibers

Ovaries

- Female gonads (homologous of testes in the male) that lie in the ovarian fossa.

- Ovarian artery (branch of the aorta) and ovarian branch of the uterine artery.

- Right ovarian vein drains into the inferior vena cava, and the left ovarian vein drains into the left renal vein.

- Pre-aortic and para-aortic lymph nodes.

- Postganglionic sympathetic (T10, T11) parasympathetic (S2, S3, and S4) fibers (Abdominal autonomic plexuses).

Vagina

- Female organ of copulation forms the lower part of the birth canal. It lies between the bladder and urethra in front and the rectum and anal canal behind. The axis of the vagina corresponds with the axis of the pelvic outlet.

- The fornix of the vagina is divided into anterior, posterior, and two lateral fornices. *Hymen of Vagina:* It is an incomplete mucous fold closing the vaginal cavity close to the external orifice of the vagina. The hymen presents various shapes—annular, crescentic, or cribriform.

- Highly vascular organ and is supplied by the vaginal artery, a branch of the internal iliac artery primarily.

- Pampiniform plexus at the vagina's sides drains through vaginal veins into the internal iliac veins.

- Internal and external, and superficial inguinal nodes.

- Sympathetic (L1, L2 spinal segments), parasympathetic (S2, S3 spinal segments) fibers, pudendal, and perineal nerve.

PATHOLOGIES

UTERUS

Case 102 Bicornuate Uterus with the Gravid Left Horn

A 28-year-old female with 5 weeks of amenorrhea (Figure 5.3).

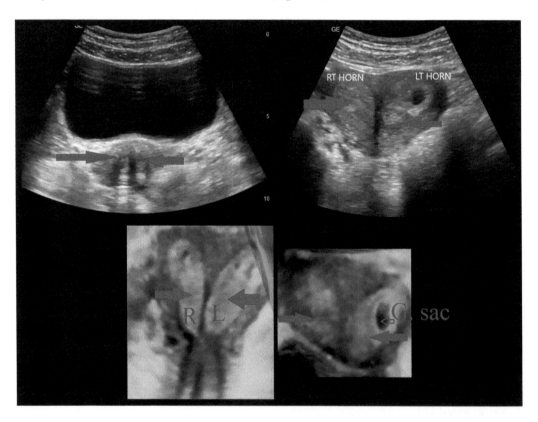

Figure 5.3 Pelvic and 3D sonography depict two separate endometrial cavities throughout the cervix with a gestational sac in the left horn.

Discussion

A bicornuate uterus is a uterine duplication anomaly due to failure of ductal fusion, usually presenting with early pregnancy loss or cervical incompetence.

Mullerian Duct Anomaly Classification (Table 5.1)

Table 5.1: **Mullerian Duct Anomalies**

1.	Mullerian agenesis	Absent/hypoplastic uterus; lacks zonal differentiation
2.	Unicornuate uterus	Banana-shaped uterus with ipsilateral fallopian tube and contralateral rudimentary horn Single normal cervix Cavitary (Communicating vs non-communicating type)
3.	Didelphys	2 Uterine horns widely separated 2 Cervix is unfused Vaginal septum present (75%)
4.	Bicornuate	2 Uterine horns widely separated (intercornual distance>4 cm) and angle>105° Concavity of fundal contour/external fundal indentation>1 cm depth 2 Cervix—unfused/fused. Myometrium extending up to internal cervical os (unicollis) or up to external cervical os (bicollis) Vaginal septum present (25%)
5.	Septate (poorest obstetrical outcome)	Convexity of fundal contour/internal indentation>1 cm depth Angle of indentation<75° Fibrous (T2 hypointense) or muscular (T2 intermediate) septum
6.	Arcuate	Minimal indentation of the myometrium into the uterine cavity Angle of indentation>90°
7.	DES-related	T-shaped uterus with narrow uterine cavity and normal cervix

Management

Recurrent pregnancy loss: Metroplasty
  Cervical incompetence: Cerclage

Case 103 Adenomyosis

A 38-year-old multiparous female with a history of menorrhagia and dysmenorrhea (Figure 5.4).

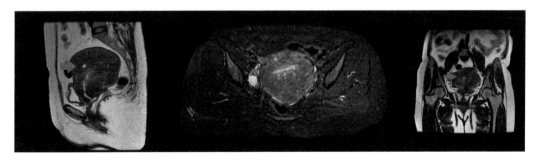

Figure 5.4   MRI reveals a bulky retroflexed uterus with a thickened junctional zone forming an ill-defined area of low signal intensity, with punctate high-intensity myometrial foci—diffuse adenomyosis.

Discussion

Adenomyosis is a benign condition marked by heterotopic basal endometrium within the myometrium a/w smooth muscle hypertrophy of the fundus and posterior wall. Patients with short menstrual cycles, early menarche, and significant estrogen exposure are more likely to develop adenomyosis. The patient presents with dyspareunia, chronic pelvic pain, menometrorrhagia, and dysmenorrhea, apart from the pelvic tenderness and diffuse enlargement of the uterus on examination. Endometriosis, leiomyomas, endometrial hyperplasia, and endometrial polyps may coexist. Adenomyosis may be generalized with preserved normal uterine contour and affects the fundus or the posterior wall of the uterus, sparing the cervix. Adenomyosis can be localized with a focal mass lesion. Cystic adenomyosis is an uncommon variant that is thought to be caused by repetitive localized hemorrhages that result in cystic areas filled with altered blood components. The normal myometrial-endometrial junction is less than 5 mm. Sonography reveals a heterogeneously enlarged uterus with indistinct endometrial-myometrial junction, asymmetric myometrial thickening (thickened sub-endometrial hypoechoic halo), myometrial cysts, and echogenic striations.

Normal zonal anatomy of the uterus on T2WI

- *Endometrium*: Hyperintense
- *Junctional Zone (JZ)*: Hypointense
- *Outer Myometrium*: Intermediate SI

MRI depicts JZ thickness due to high cellular density. Ill-defined areas of low signal intensity with myometrial and sub-endometrial cysts with thickened junctional zones up to 12 mm may be seen on MRI.

- Adenomyoma is characterized as a heterogenous ill-defined lesion (hypointense on T2WI with hyperintense tiny cystic foci) within the myometrial wall, sparing JZ and serosa.
- Accessory cavitated uterine mass (ACUM)—Nodular uterine lesion with a T1 hyperintense central cavity not connected to the endometrial cavity.

Table 5.2 differentiates between internal and external adenomyosis.

Table 5.2: **Types of Adenomyosis**

Adenomyosis	Internal	External
Location of ectopic endometrial glands	Within the internal myometrium, focal/diffuse	In the outer myometrial layers, spares JZ and involves serosa (posterior/anterior types)
Age and associations	Elderly females, prior uterine surgery history	Young, nulligravid females a/w deep infiltrating endometriosis
MRI findings	Tiny cysts/linear striations of high signal on T2WI (high signal on T1WI due to hemorrhage) JZ thickness>12 mm on sagittal T2WI	Tiny cysts of high signal on T2WI (high signal on T1WI due to hemorrhage) Bulky irregular thickening of subserosal myometrium (hypointense on T2WI)
D/D	Focal-leiomyoma, ACUM	Fibroendometriotic plaques of DIE

Pitfalls

- Preferably do scanning in the late proliferative phase and avoid during the menstrual phase as JZ is hormonal-dependent, and its thickness is maximum in the menstrual phase.
- JZ thickness reduces in pregnancy, postmenopausal females, and patients on OCPs and gonadotropins.
- Transient uterine contractions (T2 WI hypointense bands perpendicular to JZ) simulate focal adenomyosis.
- Pseudo-widening of the endometrium due to endometrial invasion of myometrium simulates endometrial carcinoma.

Differential Diagnosis

- Fibroid
- Transient uterine contraction
- Endometrial carcinoma
- Myometrial metastases

Management

- *Medical*: GnRH agonist
- *Surgical*: Hysterectomy is recommended for women for whom medical treatment does not suffice and who do not desire fertility.

Case 104 Subserosal Fibroid

A 38-year-old female with menorrhagia (Figure 5.5).

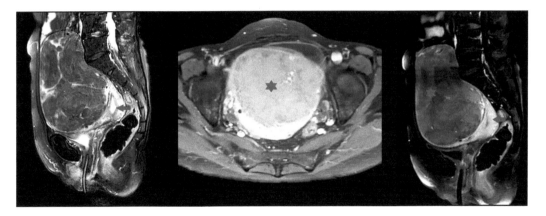

Figure 5.5 MRI abdomen depicts a large, well-defined T1 hypointense, T2 heterogeneously hypointense with postcontrast heterogeneous enhancement arising from the anterior wall of the uterus, showing multiple flow voids traversing from the uterus to the lesion.

Discussion

Uterine fibroids, leiomyomas, benign, estrogen-dependent, myometrial tumors, frequently seen in females of reproductive age group, increase in size during pregnancy and regress with menopause. Patients may be asymptomatic or may present with abnormal uterine bleeding (AUB), lower abdominal pain, infertility, etc. The pressure effect may cause urinary retention or urgency. Apart from intrauterine fibroids, they may be located in the broad ligament or cervix or wander as a parasitic leiomyoma.

Table 5.3 depicts various types of fibroids.

Table 5.3: **Types of Fibroids**

	Intramural	**Subserosal**	**Submucosal**
Frequency	Most common	Variable	Least common
Presentation	Asymptomatic, AUB	If pedunculated and torsion—acute abdomen	Most symptomatic; may prolapse
Location	Within the myometrium	Projects out from the uterus (may be pedunculated)	Projecting into the uterine cavity
Differentials	Lipoleiomyoma	Adnexal lesion	Polyps, endometrial carcinoma

Subserosal fibroids can be sessile or pedunculated. It shows vessels (flow voids on T2WI and shows contrast enhancement) coursing from the uterus into an adjoining pelvic mass, differentiating it from the adnexal mass. Fibroids may undergo torsion or prolapse.

Transvaginal sonohysterography (instillation of sterile saline via transcervical catheter into the uterine cavity) better delineates endometrium and differentiates polyp from submucosal fibroid.

On imaging, the uterus appears bulky with irregular contour and fibroids as well-circumscribed, solid hypo-/iso echoic/dense lesions with a whorled pattern exerting mass effect on the myometrium. CDUS shows peripheral vascularity, which may be absent in torsion. Fibroids are isointense on T1WI and hypointense on T2WI with variable enhancement.

Fibroids may undergo atrophy, calcification (posterior acoustic shadowing), fibrosis, and various types of changes such as hyaline (most common; hypointense T2 SI)), fatty, necrotic/cystic (hyperintense T2SI), mucoid (markedly hyperintense), and red/carneous degeneration.

Red degeneration is due to hemorrhagic infarction (venous infarction)—non-enhancing with variable signal intensity on MRI depending on the chronicity of hemorrhage. Red degeneration is noted, especially during pregnancy, and presents with acute abdominal pain. Rarely, fibroids may undergo malignant sarcomatous transformation. MRI better characterizes zonal anatomy and pelvic masses to predict and evaluate the treatment response.

Differentials

- Lipoleiomyoma (high fat content).
- Focal adenomyosis (ill-defined, no pseudo capsule, no mass effect).
- Focal myometrial contraction (repeat the sonography/MRI sequence).
- Generalized adenomyosis has a regular contour with the bulky uterus.

Management

- Hormone therapy, myomectomy/hysterectomy (depending on the age and need for future fertility)
- Uterine artery embolization (UAE)
- High-intensity focused ultrasound (HIFU)

Case 105 Endometriosis

A 29-year-old female with a history of dysmenorrhea for 3–4 years (Figure 5.6).

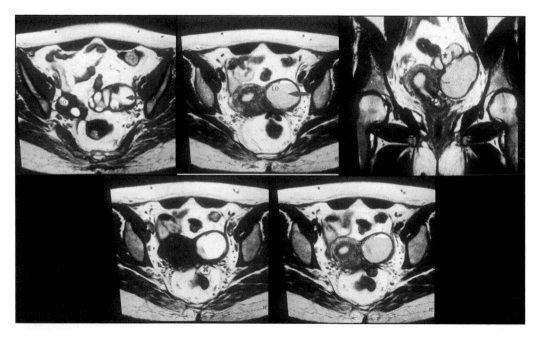

Figure 5.6 MRI pelvis depicts large and two small, well-defined T2/T1 hyperintense cystic lesions in LO with blood fluid levels and RO, respectively (bilateral endometriomas). T2/T1 hyperintense dilated tubular structure in the left adnexa (left hematosalpinx star). T2/T1 hypointense lesions within the anterior mesorectum adherent to the posterior surface of the left adnexa (fibrotic endometriotic deposits—arrowhead). Few T2/T1 hypointense bands are seen in the rectouterine pouch extending from the posterior surface of the uterus up to the ventral surface of the rectum (adhesions). A well-defined T2 intermediate/T1 hyperintense lesion within the anterior mesorectum (hemorrhagic endometriotic deposit x)—Deep endometriosis. Multiple nabothian cysts (N) in the cervix.

Discussion

Endometriosis is the development of functional ectopic endometrial glands outside the uterus—on the ovaries, fallopian tubes, bladder, ureter, rectovaginal septum, broad ligament, round ligament, and uterosacral ligament. It usually affects females of the reproductive age group and presents with chronic pelvic pain, dyspareunia, infertility, etc. It may manifest as:

- Ovarian endometriomas

- *Superficial Endometriosis*: Deposits on the surface of pelvic organs or the peritoneum, visible mainly at laparoscopy.

- Deep endometriosis with > 5 mm penetration of endometriotic lesions into retroperitoneum and adjacent visceral organs resulting in fibrous reaction and irregular solid nodules formation.

Ovarian endometriomas appear hyperintense on T1WI and hypointense on T2WI owing to cyclical bleeding. T2-Shading sign (hyperintense supernatant and hypointense dependent part) and fluid-fluid levels are characteristic signs.

Complications

Adhesions: Hypointense on T1- and T2WI fixate the bowel, pelvic organs, etc., distorting the anatomy, causing loculated fluid collections and hydrosalpinx (tortuous dilated tubular adnexal structure leading to T1 hyperintense hematosalpinx due to recurrent hemorrhages). Adhesions connecting bilateral ovaries give a 'kissing ovaries' sign. Peritubal adhesions may result in infertility.

Differentials

1. Functional hemorrhagic cysts (usually unilocular without T2 shading sign and resolve on serial examination)

2. Mucinous neoplasms (hyperintensity due to mucin is less than hemorrhage on T1WI)

3. Dermoids (contains fat; fat-saturated sequences exclude the diagnosis)

4. Abscesses (hypointense on T1WI)

5. Malignant tumors (nodularity and thick enhancing septations)

Pitfalls

- Avoid imaging during the menstrual cycle.

- The bladder should be optimally filled. Over-distended bladder results in under-diagnosis of small deposits due to obliteration of adjacent spaces and detrusor contractions. An empty bladder hinders optimum ureteral visibility.

Management

Laparoscopic surgery with tissue sampling.

Case 106 Gartner's Duct Cyst

A 39-year-old female with an incidental finding (Figure 5.7).

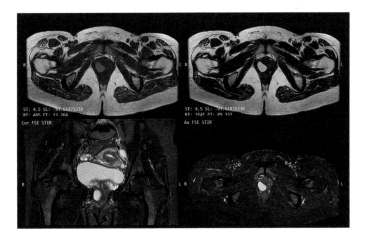

Figure 5.7 MRI pelvis depicts a thin-walled T1 hypointense, T2 hyperintense cystic lesion (not suppressing on STIR) in the right anterolateral wall of the proximal vagina just above the level of the inferior aspect of the pubic symphysis.

Discussion

Gartner's duct develops from mesonephric remnants along the anterolateral aspect of the vagina. Cysts may be found incidentally or a/w metanephric system anomalies. The typical location is above the level of pubic symphysis along the anterolateral wall of the proximal vagina.

Differentials

- Bartholin's cyst is located below the pubic symphysis level along the posterolateral vaginal wall near the introitus.

- Skene gland cysts occur due to obstructing periurethral glands and are anteriorly located at the external urethral orifice.

- Urethral diverticulum lies near the periurethral location.

All of these cysts can become infected and painful, requiring intervention.

Case 107 Skene Duct Cysts

A 5-year-old female presented with a painless lesion at the vaginal introitus (Figure 5.8).

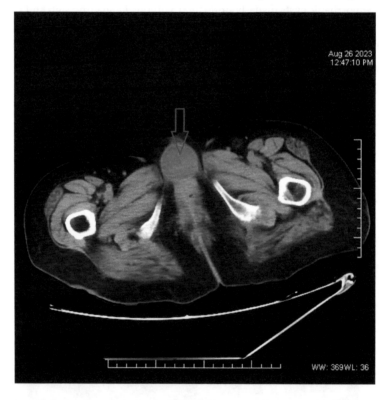

Figure 5.8 A well-defined cystic lesion in the midline caudal to the pubic symphysis and anterior to the urethra.

Discussion

Skene glands, paired paraurethral glands for lubrication, link to vaginal introitus through skene ducts duct cysts. Inflammatory blockage of the ducts with secretions forms a mass. Imaging shows a fluid density lesion, T1 hypointense, and T2 hyperintense below the pubic symphysis and posterolateral to the urethra. The lesion may be T1 intermediate/hyperintense if infected.

Differentials Diagnosis

- *Urethral Diverticulum*: Lies posterior to the urethra and shows intense peripheral enhancement.

- *Bartholin's Cyst*: Lies below the level of the pubic symphysis at the introitus.

- *Gartner's Cyst*: Lies above the level of the pubic symphysis.

Management

Surgery, if large and symptomatic.

Case 108 Uterine AVMs

A 30-year-old female with menorrhagia (Figure 5.9).

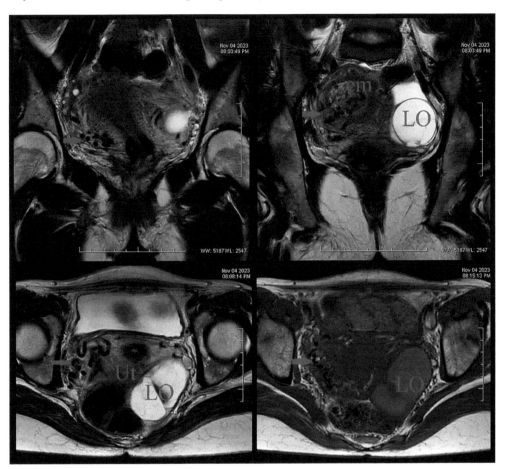

Figure 5.9 MRI pelvis depicts AV malformation (arrow) in the right broad ligament and myometrium extending to the endometrium with hemorrhagic contents in the endometrial cavity. Left ovarian hemorrhagic cyst.

Discussion

Uterine AVMs comprise multiple fistulous communications between feeding arteries and draining veins with central nidus without intervening capillary networks. It can be congenital or acquired. Acquired AVMs occur due to damage to uterine tissue due to abortion and gestational trophoblastic disease. AVMs tend to enlarge and erode into the endometrial cavity. It may be a/w miscarriages, previous surgery, and presents with heavy unexplained uterine bleeding.

Sonography depicts tubular anechoic spaces within the myometrium, prominent parametrial vessels, myometrial heterogeneity, and low-resistance, high-velocity flow patterns on CDUS. MRI reveals multiple serpentine T1 and T2 flow-related signal voids in the uterine wall, endometrial cavity, and parametrium. Contrast studies show intense enhancement and early venous return. Angiography is diagnostic.

Differentials

Increased myometrial vascularity shows a hypervascular lesion without early venous return.

Retained Products of Conception (RPOC) shows elevated b-HCG and hypervascularity mainly in the endometrial region.

Management

Medical treatment, hysteroscopic resection, and embolization.

Case 109 Uterine Rupture

A 25-year-old female post-cesarean (Figure 5.10).

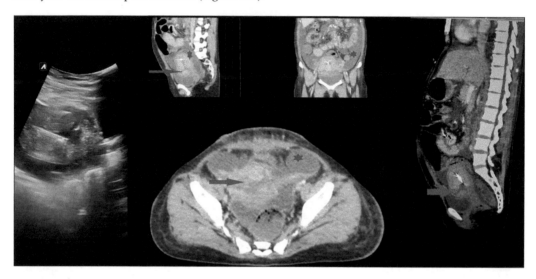

Figure 5.10 CECT abdomen depicts a mildly bulky uterus with a linear, non-enhancing hypodense tract (arrow) in the anterior myometrium in the lower uterine segment at the operative site. The tract communicates with collection (star) in the pelvic cavity, extending to the peritoneal cavity.

Discussion

Post-cesarean complications include infections, adhesions, thrombophlebitis, endometritis, wound disruption, and uterine dehiscence/rupture.

Uterine dehiscence is detached endometrium and myometrium with intact serosa compared to rupture with detachment of serosa, too, resulting in communication between uterine and peritoneal cavities with the spread of pathogenic organisms in the collection. Sonography is the initial modality of choice, though CT better delineates the hypodense tract and the extent of fluid collection.

Strategy to reduce the risk of uterine dehiscence/rupture

- Incision should be closed in two layers during surgery.
- Prevent tight interconnection of sutures that lead to ischemic necrosis.
- Use good suture material.

Management

Immediate surgery

Case 110 VVF with RVF

A 102-year-old female with a history of persistent offensive odor, recurrent vaginitis, and passage of stools through the vagina (Figure 5.11).

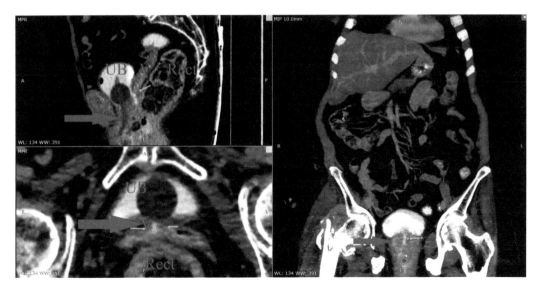

Figure 5.11 CT depicts fistulous communication between the urinary bladder and anterior vaginal wall and the posterior vaginal wall and rectum.

Discussion

Vesicovaginal fistula (VVF) refers to fistulous communication between the posterior wall of the urinary bladder and the anterior vaginal wall. Patients frequently present with recurrent UTIs and incontinence. Rectovaginal fistulas refer to fistulous communication between the anterior wall of the rectum and the posterior vaginal wall, with the passage of flatus and stool through the vagina and a history of recurrent resistant vaginitis as clinical presentation.

These fistulas are relatively rare in developed countries and common in developing and under-developed countries, the notable etiologies being obstetric or surgical trauma, infections, malignancies (cervical cancer), inflammatory diseases (Crohn's disease, diverticulitis), foreign body irritation, and post-radiotherapy.

Usually, proctography and vaginography were available initially. Methylene blue instilled into the rectum may discern a vaginal communication, but CT-vaginography is being used these days for demonstrating the communication. Localized interruption of the hypointense vaginal muscularis and the bladder wall with fistulous communication is better appreciated on T2WI with hyperintense urine and hypointense gas bubbles.

Management

The surgical (open/laparoscopic/robotic) approach depends on the site of the fistula and the presence of active underlying disease. Fistula repair with flap interposition in the same operation/staged repair can be planned.

Case 111 Iatrogenic Ureteric Injury Post-Hysterectomy

A 38-year-old female with a history of total abdominal hysterectomy (TAH) (Figure 5.12).

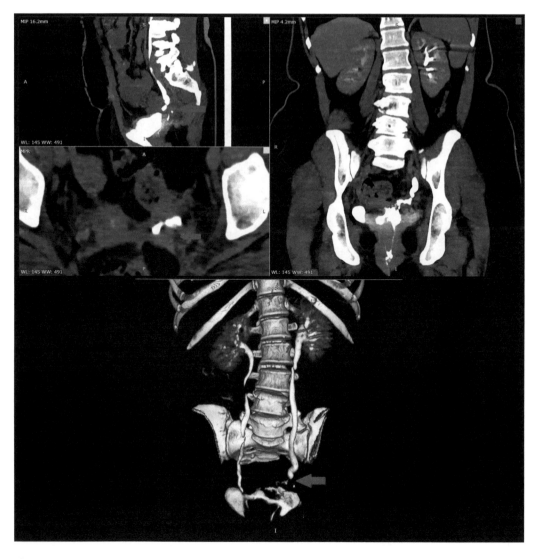

Figure 5.12 CT urography with volume rendering depicts a complete cut-off (approximately 20 mm defect) of the distal ureter up to VUJ with focal extravasation of contrast excretion from the left distal ureter extending into the vaginal cavity through the vaginal cuff.

Discussion

Iatrogenic urinary tract injuries represent widely recognized, potentially hazardous complications after gynecologic surgeries, especially TAH. The most frequent cause of ureterovaginal fistulae is a surgical injury to the distal ureter; the common risk factors are progressive cancer, diabetes, obesity, prior surgery, adhesions, and radiation. CT/MR urography plays a pivotal role in assessing postoperative complications, and delayed imaging (5–20 minutes after intravenous contrast) should be done in every patient after gynecologic surgery.

Management

Stent placement

Case 112 Tamoxifen-Induced Endometrial Hyperplasia

A 65-year-old female on tamoxifen therapy underwent CT to rule out metastasis (Figure 5.13).

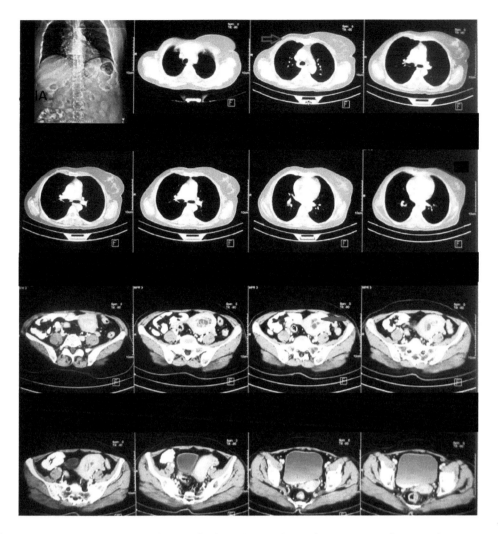

Figure 5.13   CECT abdomen depicts thickened irregular endometrium with cystic changes in a patient with a right mastectomy.

Discussion

Tamoxifen is a non-steroidal selective estrogen receptor modulator (SERM). Patients with carcinoma breast who are treated with tamoxifen may develop endometrial hyperplasia irregularity with cystic changes. Patients may present with AUB.

Normal endometrium measures <5 mm.

Management

- *Asymptomatic Patients*: No further evaluation.

- *Premenopausal Women with Amenorrhea*: Expectant management.

- *Postmenopausal Women with Vaginal Bleeding/Discharge*: To rule out endometrial cancer by transvaginal ultrasound and biopsy.

Case 113 Endometrial Carcinoma

A 56-year-old female with postmenopausal bleeding (Figure 5.14).

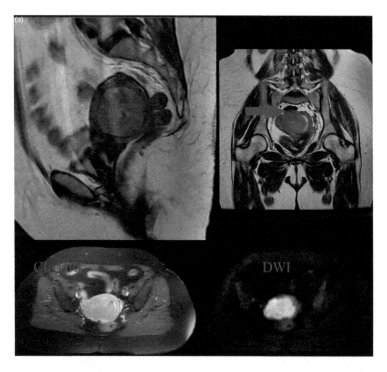

Figure 5.14 MRI pelvis, depicts a heterogeneously enhancing lesion (star) in the endometrial cavity with loss of endo-myometrial junction and serosal infiltration (arrow) on the right side. Restricted diffusion is seen on DWI.

Discussion

Endometrial carcinoma predominantly affects menopausal and postmenopausal females with associated risk factors, such as estrogen treatment, tamoxifen, obesity, nulliparity, genetic suscepti-bility, diabetes, polycystic ovaries, etc.

Histological types and Staging of endometrial carcinoma (Tables 5.4 and 5.5).

Table 5.4: **Histological Types of Endometrial Carcinoma**

Type 1	Type 2
Endometrioid adenocarcinoma, more common	Clear-cell, serous-papillary, and sarcomatous types; less common
a/w hyperestrogenism, obesity	Not a/w high estrogen
Low-grade; good prognosis	Poor prognosis

Table 5.5: **Staging of Endometrial Carcinoma**

0.	Carcinoma In Situ
1.	Limited to the uterus (with endocervix)
	a. < Half myometrial invasion
	b. > Half myometrial invasion
2.	Cervix stroma invasion
3.	Extension outside the uterus
	a. Uterine serosa
	b. Vaginal/parametrial
	c. Pelvic or para-aortic lymph nodes
4.	a. Bladder/bowel involvement
	b. Distant spread

Sonography, especially TVUS, depicts heterogeneous polypoidal/irregular endometrial thickening (< 5 mm cut-off for postmenopausal females), infiltrating the myometrium by breaching sub endometrial hypoechoic halo. Saline distension during sonohysterography evaluates the endometrium better. The lesion is hypodense and less enhancing on CT. MRI better delineates the myometrial invasion, extrauterine extent, and lymph node evaluation. T2WI shows hyperintense thickened endometrium, discontinuous hypointense junctional zone, and hyperintense cervical stromal invasion apart from differentiating the lesion, especially in patients with coexisting fibroids. Heterogeneous contrast enhancement and restricted diffusion may be seen. Endometrial biopsy is confirmative.

Pitfalls

■ Myometrial thinning in postmenopausal elderly females/coexisting fibroids should be considered while assessing for myometrial invasion.

■ Isointense tumors, mucinous tumors, and tumors positioned in the cornua make it challenging to assess myometrial invasion.

Differentials

■ Submucosal fibroids

■ Endometrial polyps

■ Other malignancies, such as carcinoma cervix infiltrating into the endometrium

■ Cystic hyperplasia due to tamoxifen therapy

Management

TAH with bilateral salpingo-oophorectomy (fertility is not required) +/– chemo/radiotherapy, depending on the stage and invasion.

Case 114 Endometrial Carcinoma with Fundal Fibroid

A 61-year-old female with postmenopausal bleed.

Discussion—Last case

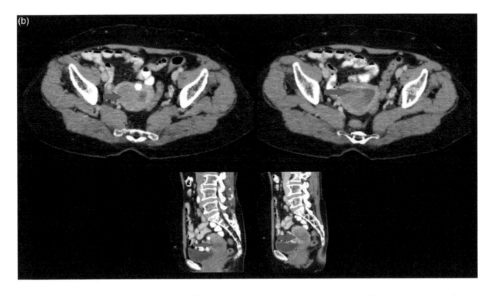

Figure 5.14   (b) CECT pelvis depicts heterogeneously enhancing mass in the endometrial cavity infiltrating uterine myometrium with a calcified fundal fibroid.

Case 115 Carcinoma Cervix 2B

A 48-year-old female with vaginal bleeding for 3 months (Figure 5.15).

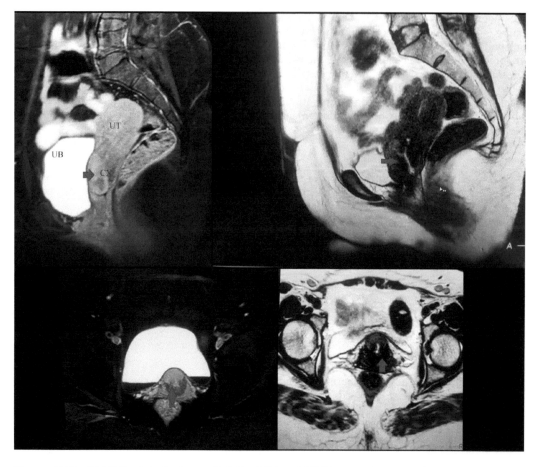

Figure 5.15 (a) MRI pelvis depicts well-defined T1 and T2W intermediate signal intensity lesion in the anterior cervix extending into the upper third of the vagina with parametrial invasion (disruption of hypointense serosal rim)—stage 2B.

Discussion

Squamous cell carcinoma is the most common histological type arising from the squamocolumnar junction. Adenocarcinoma is the less common type, mainly involving the endocervix.

Carcinoma cervix is frequent in females with young age at first intercourse, multiple sexual partners, smokers, poor hygiene, HPV 16,18, immunosuppression, etc. Patients may present with abnormal bleeding and discharge.

Sonography depicts heterogeneously hypoechoic mass with increased vascularity. MRI is better in delineating to assess the parametrial invasion and extent into adjacent organs apart from hydronephrosis. The parametrium constitutes fat, lymphatics, and vessels between the uterine body and the pelvic sidewall. CT/PET scan depicts lymphadenopathy and distant spread. Normal cervical stroma is hypointense. Carcinoma cervix appears isointense on T1WI and hyperintense on T2WI with heterogeneous contrast enhancement.

Nodal involvement

1. *Obturator Nodes (Lateral Pelvic Side Walls)*: Sentinel nodes

2. External iliac lymph nodes (extension into parametrium and pelvic side walls)

3. Inguinal nodes (extension into the lower third of the vagina)

4. Inferior mesenteric and para-aortic nodes (extension into the rectum)

Tumor spread (Table 5.6)

Table 5.6: **Staging of Carcinoma Cervix**

Cis	Carcinoma In Situ (Preinavsive)
T1	Confined to uterus
	a. < 5 mm (microscopic) b. > 4 cm (clinically visible)
T2	Extends beyond the uterus (not to lower vagina and pelvic side wall)
	a. Without parametrial invasion b. With parametrial invasion
T3	Lymph Node involvement +/−
	a. Extends to the lower third of the vagina b. Extends to pelvic side wall with hydronephrosis
T4	Invades bladder, rectum
Regional LAP	Absent (N0) or present (N1)
Distant metastasis	Absent (M0) or present (M1)

Differentials

- Lesions such as polyps, fibroids, etc., primarily involve the cervix

- Lesions such as endometrial or vaginal malignancies infiltrating into the cervix

- Metastasis to cervix

Pitfalls

- Reactive changes after biopsy exaggerate the size and extent of parametrial invasion.

- Before doing an MRI, precaution should be taken to get the bladder and rectum evacuated at least half an hour before the scan for optimal position of the uterus to avoid image degradation from an overfilled/empty urinary bladder or loaded rectum.

Management

Depends on histologic grading and tumor staging

- Surgery with chemo/radiotherapy for stages 1 and 2a.

- 2a vs. 2b differentiates the operability of the tumor.

Trachelectomy preserves fertility (cervix removal with uterovaginal anastomosis)

Case 116 Advanced Carcinoma Cervix with Hydroureteronephrosis

A 52-year-old female k/c/o carcinoma cervix (post chemo/radiotherapy).
   Discussion (Last case)

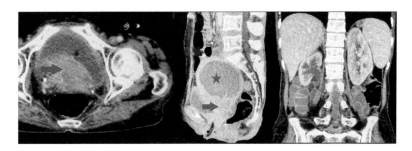

Figure 5.15   (b) CECT abdomen depicts a bulky cervix with an ill-defined heterogeneously enhancing hypodense mass (arrow) arising from the anterior lip, extending into the upper two-thirds of the vagina, causing obliteration of the endometrial canal leading to gross hypodense collection (star) in the endometrial cavity with infiltration of the posterior wall and bladder neck encasing distal ureter with right hydroureteronephrosis (arrowhead). Multiple small mesenteric, internal iliac, and para-aortic lymph nodes. Bilateral tubal ligation falope rings (open arrows).

OVARIES

Case 117 Ovarian Dermoid

A 32-year-old female on routine sonography.

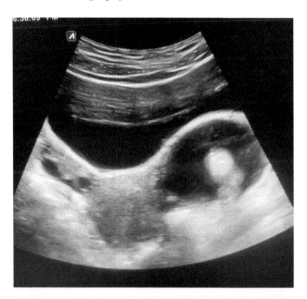

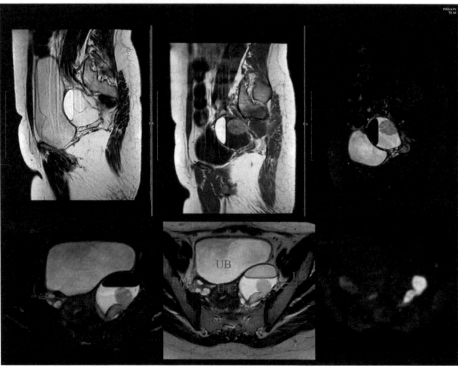

Figure 5.16 (a) Sonography reveals a unilocular echogenic lesion with an echogenic nodule in the left ovary. (b) MRI axial and sagittal views depict an enlarged left ovary with nodular components, fat-fluid level, and restricted diffusion. The right ovary (open arrow) appears normal with multiple follicles. (c) CT from another patient showing a fat density lesion with Rokitansky protuberance in the right ovary.

(Continued)

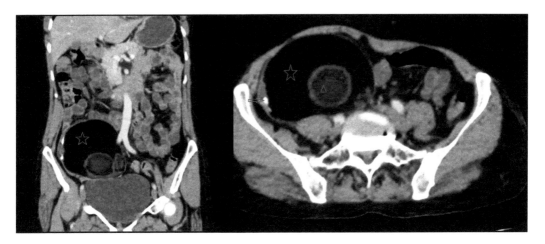

Figure 5.16 (*Continued*) Sonography reveals a unilocular echogenic lesion with an echo-genic nodule in the left ovary. (b) MRI axial and sagittal views depict an enlarged left ovary with nodular components, fat-fluid level, and restricted diffusion. The right ovary (open arrow) appears normal with multiple follicles. (c) CT from another patient showing a fat density lesion with Rokitansky protuberance in the right ovary.

Discussion

Ovarian teratomas

1. Mature cystic teratoma (dermoid)

2. Immature teratomas

3. Monodermal tumors (specialized such as struma ovarii)

The tumors are usually asymptomatic, slow-growing, discovered incidentally, and common in young females. The lesions may be complicated to ovarian torsion/rupture and present with acute pelvic pain or transform into malignancy if the size is >10 cm with irregular borders.

Sonography reveals diffusely or partially echogenic unilocular lesions with varied patterns due to fat, hair, hyperechoic Rokitansky nodule (Figure 5.16), calcific tooth, and fat-fluid levels. The lesion is avascular on CDUS. CT corroborates diagnosis with characteristic fat attenuation (negative HU) within the cyst. MRI depicts a hyperintense signal due to fat on T1- and T2WI with suppression of fat on fat-saturated T1WI. Chemical shift artifacts can confirm the presence of fat. Contrast-enhanced images are unnecessary and mainly used to recognize solid invasive components with the staging of malignant variety.

Differential Diagnosis

1. Hemorrhagic ovarian cyst

2. Ovarian serous/mucinous cystadenoma

3. Endometrioma (T2 shading and high T1SI that does not suppress with fat saturation sequences)

Management

■ Observation for small-size lesions.

■ Follow-up to monitor growth and surgery for larger lesions.

Case 118 Bilateral Tubo-Ovarian Masses

A 25-year-old female with fever, nausea, and pelvic pain (Figure 5.17).

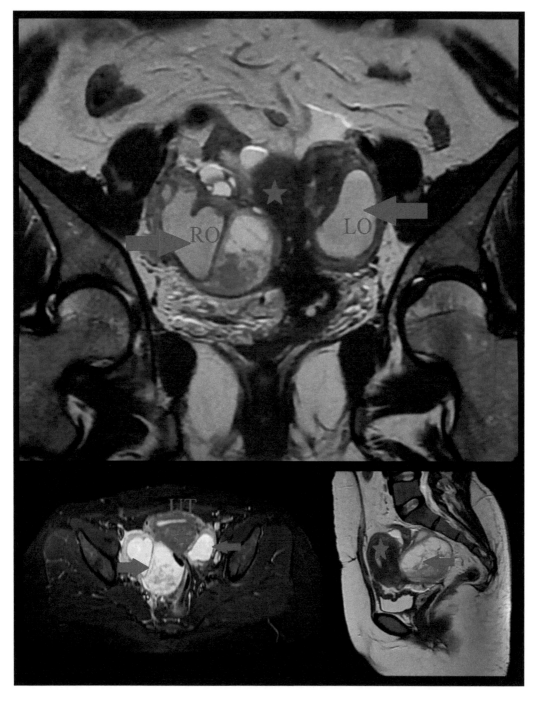

Figure 5.17 MRI pelvis depicts multiloculated collections involving bilateral adnexal region involving the ovaries.

Discussion

A tubo-ovarian abscess (TOA), a polymicrobial infection that spreads from the lower genital tract in females of the reproductive age group, is a grave complication of acute pelvic inflammatory disease (PID). The risk factors include multiple sexual partners, use of intrauterine devices, prior incidents of PID, diabetes, immunosuppression, lower socioeconomic status, and poor hygiene. Patients may present with lower abdominal pain, fever, discharge, nausea, etc. PID may be a/w perihepatitis, resulting in Fitz-Hugh-Curtis syndrome. It may be caused by anaerobic bacteria such as Bacteroides, actinomycosis (more solid than cystic), tuberculosis (usually a/w peritoneal involvement), etc. The lesions may rupture, involve the colon, ureter, etc., causing respective symptoms. Infertility or ectopic pregnancy are late complications.

Sonography reveals bilateral multiloculated, irregularly thick-walled, complex solid cystic, adnexal masses with septations and echogenic debris. CECT shows heterogeneously enhancing lesions with fluid-fluid levels or air pockets, thickened uterosacral ligaments, adjacent fat stranding, and ascites. The lesions appear hypointense on T1WI and heterogeneously hyperintense on T2WI, depending on the proteinaceous content and viscosity of the lesion.

Differentials

- Hemorrhagic cysts (High signal on T1- and T2WI)
- Endometriomas
- Abscesses due to other causes such as Crohn's disease, diverticulitis, etc.
- Hydrosalpinx
- Broad ligament leiomyomas.
- Peritoneal inclusion cysts
- Benign ovarian tumors, such as teratomas
- Ovarian malignancy
- Ovarian metastasis (Krukenberg's tumor)

Management

Antibiotics, image-guided drainage

Case 119 Ruptured Ectopic

A 25-year-old female with unstable hemodynamics (Figure 5.18).

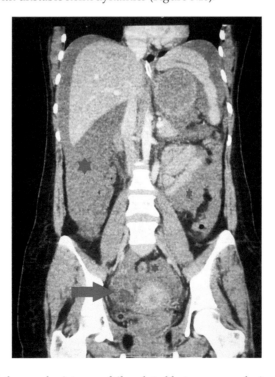

Figure 5.18   CECT abdomen depicts a multiloculated heterogenous lesion in the right adnexa (arrow) and gross hemoperitoneum (star).

Discussion

Ectopic pregnancy refers to blastocyst implantation outside the uterine endometrium. Heterotopic pregnancy occurs as ectopic with co-existent intrauterine pregnancy. Sonography is the modality of choice for diagnosing ectopic pregnancy, along with a positive hCG test. The classic triad of ectopic pregnancy constitutes severe abdominal pain, vaginal bleeding, and tender adnexal mass and is the pivotal cause of high maternal mortality. Ruptured ectopic pregnancy usually presents with hemodynamic instability with hypotension, tachycardia, reducing hematocrit, and rebound tenderness. Imaging shows ruptured ectopic as a multiloculated complex adnexal lesion with gross hemoperitoneum in the peritoneal and pelvic cavities.

Pitfalls

Suspect ectopic pregnancy in any female in the reproductive age group presenting with acute abdominal pain. CT is usually not required and may be performed unintentionally, as the pain mimics other causes of acute abdomen, such as appendicitis, diverticulitis, etc. hCG testing is mandatory.

Management

Immediate laparotomy

Case 120 Recurrent Ovarian Tumor with Metastasis

K/C/O bilateral papillary serous cystadenocarcinoma (postoperative status) (Figure 5.19).

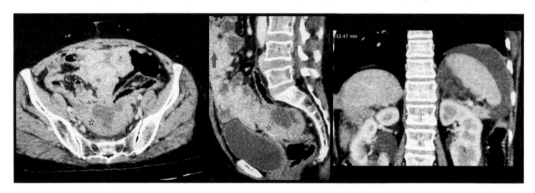

Figure 5.19   CECT abdomen depicts a large, ill-defined, lobulated heterogeneously enhancing solid cystic lesion (star) in the pelvic cavity predominantly on the right side with loss of fat planes with adjacent bowel loops, urinary bladder, and right lower ureter causing mild right hydroureteronephrosis. Omental fat shows extensive fat stranding and nodularities (Omental caking) (solid arrow). Multiple ill-defined heterogeneously enhancing hypodense lesions along peritoneal lining in bilateral subdiaphragmatic, perigastric, and bilateral paracolic space with enhancing nodular peritoneal lining—likely peritoneal deposits (arrowhead). Moderate ascites (circle).

Discussion

Ovarian carcinomas mostly present with abdominopelvic pain, abdominal fullness, and mass lesions. The risk factors include smoking, obesity, nulliparity, gonadal dysgenesis, early menarche, late menopause, family history, especially with *BRCA1/BRCA2* mutations, and Lynch syndrome. Breastfeeding and oral contraceptive pills (OCP) are considered protective.

Table 5.7 shows general classification of ovarian tumors.

Table 5.7: **General Classification of Ovarian Tumors**

General Subtypes	Further Categories
Surface epithelial-stromal tumors	• Serous cystadenomas/carcinomas • Mucinous cystadenomas/carcinomas • Endometroid tumor • Clear cell type • Brenner tumor • Squamous cell carcinoma
Germ cell tumors (GCTs)	• Teratoma (mature/immature/specialized-struma ovarii types) • Yolk sac (endodermal sinus tumors) • Dysgerminoma • Embryonal cell tumor • Choriocarcinoma
Sex-cord/stromal tumors	• Sertoli-Leydig cell tumor • Ovarian fibroma • Ovarian thecoma • Granulosa cell tumor (juvenile/adult type) • Sclerosing stromal
Lymphoma Sarcoma	
Metastases	• Krukenberg tumors • Others

Epithelial tumors with cystic-solid components and distinctive papillary projections can be invasive or noninvasive. Brenner's tumor is mostly benign. The criteria for malignancy include cystic-solid nature, size greater than 4 cm, thick, irregular wall and septa, papillary projections, necrosis, and neoangiogenesis. Ovarian malignancies are usually associated with ascites and peritoneal carcinomatosis. Sometimes, the cyst may rupture, leading to pseudomyxoma peritonei with thick mucinous material in the peritoneal cavity and scalloping of surfaces of the liver and spleen. Transabdominal and endovaginal sonography are used initially to detect the lesion. CECT is important in evaluating the spread of malignant lesions and in detecting recurrence after therapy. MRI is better at characterizing the adnexal mass and detecting the local spread. *18 F-FDG PET/CT* is beneficial in postoperative follow-up patients with suspected recurrence.

Staging of ovarian tumors (Table 5.8)

Table 5.8: **Staging of Ovarian Tumors**

Stage	Localization
1.	Ovaries
2.	Extension to pelvis (contralateral ovary, uterus, and fallopian tubes)
3.	Intraperitoneal dissemination, ascites, and lymph nodes
4.	Distant metastasis to liver, spleen, pleural effusion, etc

Tumor serum markers such as cancer antigen (CA)-125 are better in postmenopausal women, while Human epididymis protein 4 (HE4) aids in differentiating benign and malignant adnexal masses in premenopausal women.

Differential Diagnosis

Recurrent Lesions

■ Postoperative hematomas

■ Postoperative bacterial peritonitis (diffuse peritoneal thickening)

■ Chemical peritonitis in patients with intraperitoneal chemotherapy

Adnexal Lesions

■ Different subtypes of ovarian neoplasms

■ Hydro/pyo/hematosalpinx

- Fallopian tube cancer
- Endometriosis
- Metastases

Management

TAH with bilateral salpingo-oophorectomy (BSO) +/– chemotherapy in primary tumors. Secondary cytoreduction in cases of recurrence.

Case 121 Krukenberg's Tumor

A 40-year-old female k/c/o gastric malignancy (signet ring cell type) (Figure 5.20).

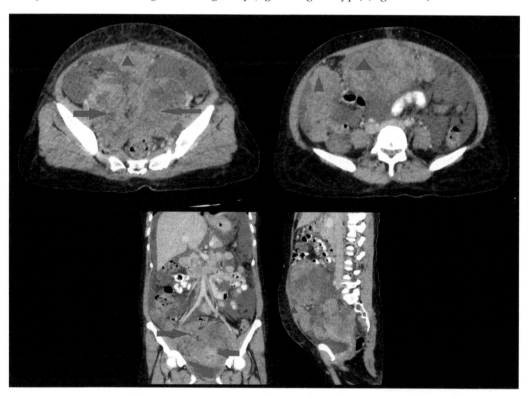

Figure 5.20 CECT abdomen depicts large, ill-defined multilobulated complex hypoattenuating solid cystic lesions showing heterogenous enhancement in bilateral adnexa (arrows) showing loss of fat planes with fundus and posterior wall of uterus, anterior wall of upper and mid rectum, bilateral external and internal iliac arteries and bilateral psoas muscle. Multiple enlarged, ill-defined, heterogeneously enhancing soft tissue lesions along the parietal peritoneum, omentum, right ileocolic region, and peritoneal and pelvic cavity (peritoneal dissemination—arrowhead—metastatic deposits). Gross ascites (star).

Discussion

Krukenberg's tumor is a metastatic tumor to ovaries by a mucin-secreting signet ring cell adeno-carcinoma from primary malignancy in stomach, colon, pancreaticobiliary, or appendix. They are frequent in young females owing to the propensity of functioning ovaries with rich blood supply to metastatic disease. Patients present with irregular vaginal bleeding, dyspareunia, bloating, pelvic pain, etc.

Imaging shows bilateral heterogeneously enhancing solid cystic adnexal lesions (bosselated/bumpy conour0 with interspersed hyperechoic/dense areas (due to mucin), hypoechoic/dense regions (due to fibrosis), and moth-eaten cyst formation. Solid areas are hypointense on T1- and T2WI due to dense ovarian stroma and interspersed hyperintense cystic areas containing mucin.

Abundant lymphatics draining gastric mucosa and submucosa initiate retrograde lymphatic spread to the ovary.

Differentials

- *Primary Epithelial Ovarian Malignancy*: Common in elderly females > 55 years

- Peritoneal carcinomatosis due to ovarian malignancy

- Bilateral endometriomas, dermoids, and hemorrhagic cysts. (signal intensity difference depending upon the content)

- Ovarian hyperstimulation stimulation syndrome (especially in females undergoing infertility treatment)

- Bilateral tubo-ovarian abscesses

- Bilateral solid tumors such as fibromas, thecomas, Brenner tumors, etc.

Management

Poor prognosis

PEDIATRICS

Case 122 Mayer-Rokitansky-Küster-Hauser (MRKH) Syndrome

A late-adolescent female with primary amenorrhea and normal hormonal levels (Figure 5.21).

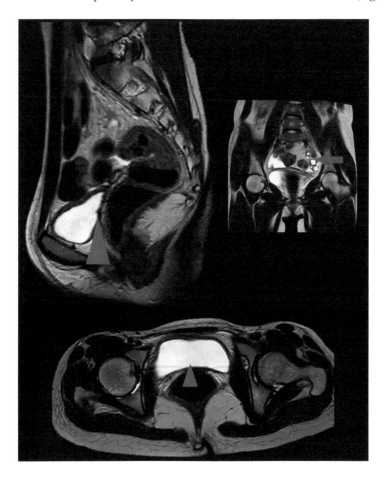

Figure 5.21 MRI pelvis depicts an empty uterine bed (arrowhead) between the bladder and rectum with agenesis of the uterus, cervix, and proximal vagina with T1- and T2 hypointense rudimentary vaginal stump in the rectovesical pouch. Bilateral normal ovaries (arrow).

Discussion

Arrested development of the paramesonephric ducts, during embryogenesis, at approximately 7 weeks after fertilization, results in the underdevelopment of the uterus and upper two-thirds of the vagina but normal ovaries, fallopian tubes, and external genitalia (classic type A MRKH). Associated abnormalities of the Mullerian system (ovaries, fallopian tubes), renal, and spine are part of the atypical form of MRKH (type B). It presents with normal hormonal levels and an external phenotype with 46 XX karyotypes. Ovarian follicles appear hyperintense, and stroma appears hypointense on T2WI. HSG is the initial imaging modality to assess tubal patency and evaluate for infertility. Sonohysterography with saline infusion, 3D sonography, and MRI better depict endometrium and uterine morphology.

Differentials

Androgen insensitive syndrome—Virilization of external genitalia resulting in the development of female secondary sexual characteristics and genotypically male (46XY) with undescended testes.

Management

Vaginal dilatation or creation of neovagina/vaginoplasty.
  Psychological counseling

Case 123 Gonadal Dysgenesis with Mullerian Agenesis

A short-stature female with primary amenorrhea (Figure 5.22).

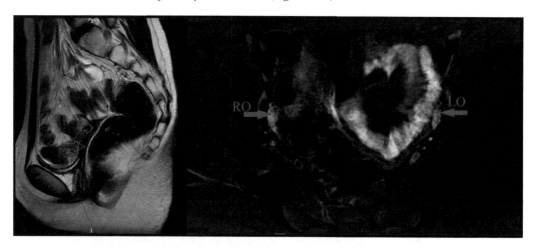

Figure 5.22 MR pelvis depicts bilateral hypoplastic streak ovaries at the lateral pelvic wall and hypoplastic uterus with a thin strip of the vagina (arrows).

Discussion

MRKH features with the absence of a uterus, fallopian tubes, and upper two-thirds of the vagina (s/o hypoestrogenic state) with bilateral streak ovaries due to stromal fibrosis (without follicles) in an ectopic location (lateral pelvic wall) suggests Turner's syndrome. TS is a form of gonadal dysgenesis with a chromosomal disorder (XO) with partial or complete absence of the X chromosome; common in females with streak ovaries with primary amenorrhea or premature ovarian failure. Patients have normal intelligence and may show a webbed neck, low hairline at the back, lymphoedema of hand and foot, skeletal abnormalities (short 4th metacarpal, scoliosis), horseshoe kidney, and coarctation of aorta.

Management

- Hormonal therapy (to develop secondary sexual characters)
- Very little chance of conception

Case 124 Septate Uterus with Right Hematocolpos

A 15-year-old female with heavy menstrual bleeding for 2 months (Figure 5.23).

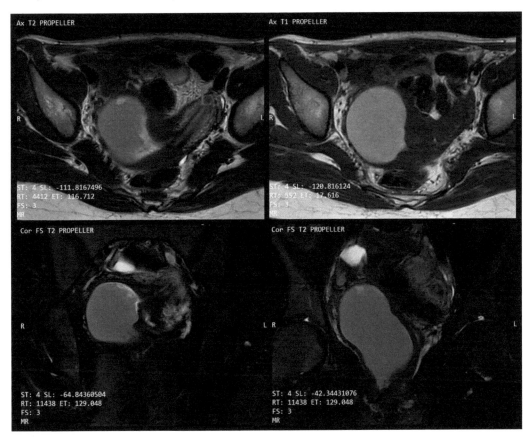

Figure 5.23 MRI pelvis depicts two separate uterine cavities with two cervices and two vaginas, divided by a T2 hypointense longitudinal septum extending up to the cervix. Grossly distended right vaginal cavity with T1 hyperintense and T2 intermediate collection-hematocolpos.

Discussion

Septate uterus occurs due to failure of resorption of the uterine septum at approximately the 20th week of gestation. Septate uterus increases the risk of early pregnancy loss and subfertility. Subseptate uterus with partial septum involves endometrial cavity and spares cervix.

Discussed in Case 1

Management

Hysteroscopic resection of septum

Case 125 OHVIRA (Obstructed HemiVagina, Ipsilateral Renal Agenesis)

A 15-year-old female presented with lower abdominal pain for 4 months. Menarche at 14 years with a normal menstrual cycle (Figure 5.24).

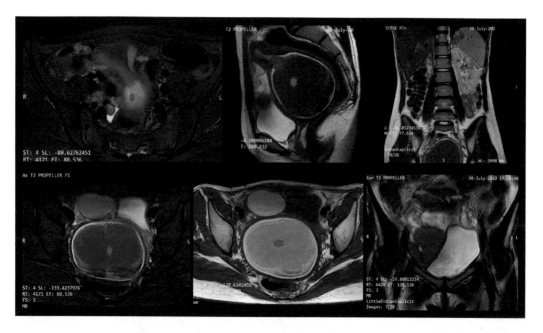

Figure 5.24 MRI abdomen reveals a developmentally malformed uterus with two separate endometrial cavities (arrows) and a complete septum extending into the cervix. Markedly dilated right-sided endometrial and cervical cavity with hemorrhagic collection—hematometra (star). Hematosalpinx and absent right kidney.

Discussion

OHVIRA, also known as Herlyn–Werner–Wunderlich Syndrome (HWWS), is rare and presents as a triad of obstructed hemivagina, ipsilateral renal agenesis, and uterine didelphys resulting in hematometrocolpos. It occurs due to the lateral non-fusion of the Mullerian ducts with obstruction.

The normal menses from unobstructed hemivagina simulate a normal menstrual cycle, and hence, the patient presents late, usually with abdominal pain, dysmenorrhea, pelvic mass, infertility, spontaneous abortion, etc. The retrograde flow of menstrual products through the obstructed outflow tract may result in endometriosis. The counterpart of OHVIRA in males is OSVIRA, discussed in Chapter 3. Sonography reveals a large cystic lesion with low-level echoes in the pelvic cavity with ipsilateral absent kidney and uterine didelphys though it's difficult to visualize the vaginal septum, which is better delineated on MRI.

Differentials

Hematometrocolopos should be differentiated from hemorrhagic adnexal masses, especially on sonography.

Management

Vaginoplasty +/– metroplasty

SUGGESTED READINGS

Behr, S. C., Courtier, J. L., & Qayyum, A. Imaging of Müllerian duct anomalies. *RadioGraphics* 2012;32:6, E233–E250.

Drake, R. L., & Vogl, A. W. (2020). *Gray's Atlas of Anatomy E-Book*. Elsevier Health Sciences.

Jung, S. E., Lee, J. M., Rha, S. E., Byun, J. Y., Jung, J. I., & Hahn, S. T. CT and MR imaging of ovarian tumors with emphasis on differential diagnosis. *RadioGraphics* 2002;22:6, 1305–1325.

Lee, J., & Sagel, T. (2006). *Computed Body Tomography with MRI Correlation*. Lippincott Williams & Wilkins.

Lumley, J. S., & Craven, J. L. (2018). *Bailey & Love's Essential Clinical Anatomy*. CRC Press.

Otero-García, M. M., Mesa-Álvarez, A., Nikolic, O. et al. Role of MRI in staging and follow-up of endometrial and cervical cancer: Pitfalls and mimickers. *Insights Imaging* 2019;10:19. doi: 10.1186/s13244-019-0696-8.

Saleh, M. Cervical cancer: 2018 revised international federation of gynecology and obstetrics staging system and the role of imaging. *Am J Radiol*. 2017;214(5). doi: 10.2214/AJR.19.21819.

6 Male Pelvic System

EMBRYOLOGY

Development of Scrotum and Testis

The scrotum develops from labioscrotal swellings and urogenital folds, which fuse in the midline to form the scrotum. The testis develops from the genital ridge of the developing mesonephros at the level of the T10 segment.

- *Mesonephric Tubules*: Efferent ductules of the testis.

- *Mesonephric Duct*: Duct of epididymis, vas deferens, seminal vesicles (diverticulum from the caudal part), and ejaculatory duct.

- *Embryological Remnants*: Appendix of (testis and epididymis), paradidymis, and superior and inferior aberrant ductules.

Development of Prostate

- *Glandular Portion*: The pelvic part of the urogenital sinus forms solid endodermal outgrowths, which canalize to form follicles and ductules of the gland (third month of intrauterine life).

- Fibromuscular part of the gland develops from the splanchnic mesoderm surrounding the urogenital sinus (fourth month of intrauterine life) (Figure 6.1).

ANATOMY

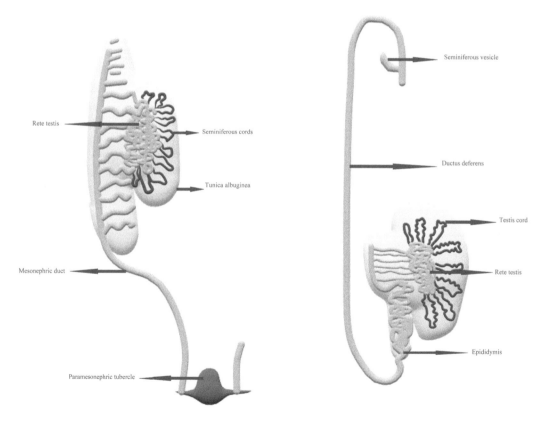

Figure 6.1 Development of the male reproductive system.

The male genital organs are classified into two: external and internal.
 The external genital organs include the following structures:

Penis

- Male organ of copulation, traversed by the urethra, passage for urine and semen.
- Root of the penis is situated in the superficial perineal pouch.
- Three masses of erectile tissue, viz., two crura and the bulb of the penis.
- Body of the penis is the free pendulous portion which lies in front of the scrotum and terminates in the glans penis. It comprises three (two corpora cavernosa and one corpus spongiosum) elongated masses of erectile tissue, which are capable of considerable enlargement when engorged with blood during an erection.
- Six pairs of arteries (the first three pairs of arteries arise from *internal pudendal arteries,* and the last pair arises from *superficial external pudendal arteries*, branches of femoral arteries).
- Superficial dorsal vein of the penis drains into the external pudendal vein, and the deep dorsal vein of the penis drains into the prostatic venous plexus.
- Deep inguinal lymph nodes, especially into the lymph node of cloquet and superficial inguinal lymph nodes.
- Sensory innervation is by the dorsal nerve of the penis and the ilioinguinal nerve; motor innervation is the perineal branch of the pudendal nerve, and autonomic innervation: pelvic (inferior hypogastric) plexus via the prostatic plexus.

Scrotum

- Large pendulous sac of skin located below and behind the penis
- Divided into right and left halves by a median ridge or raph
- Skin is dark and rugose (corrugated) due to the presence of subcutaneous dartos muscle)
- Superficial and deep external pudendal arteries, scrotal branches of the internal pudendal artery, and cremasteric artery from the inferior epigastric artery
- Superficial inguinal lymph nodes
- Ilioinguinal nerve, genital branch of genitofemoral nerve (L1) and perineal nerve (S3)

Testis

- Male gonad, that produces spermatozoa and secretes testosterone hormone.
- It is suspended in the scrotum by the spermatic cord.
- It is enclosed in a fibrous capsule, the *tunica albuginea.*
- Posteriorly, it is thickened to form an incomplete vertical septum/ridge, the *mediastinum testis.*
- Numerous fibrous septa extend from the mediastinum to the inner aspect of the tunica albuginea and divide the interior of the testis into 200–300 lobules.
- Each lobule contains 2–4 coiled seminiferous tubules lined by thick multilayered germinal epithelium that produces spermatozoa. The thin, thread-like loops of seminiferous tubules join each other and become straighter as they pass toward the mediastinum, forming straight *tubules, then form a* network of channels called the *rete testis.* The small *efferent ductules* connect the rete testis channels to the epididymis's upper end. The interstitial cells lie in the areolar tissue between the seminiferous tubules.
- Testicular artery (L2)
- Pampiniform plexus of veins
- Pre-aortic and Para-aortic groups of lymph nodes
- Sympathetic nerves (T10)

Epididymis

- Comma-shaped structure on the superior and posterolateral surface of the testis.

- Made up of highly coiled tubes that act as a reservoir of spermatozoa.

- Divided into the head (highly coiled efferent ductules) and body and tail (single highly coiled duct of epididymis).

Spermatic Cord

- Constitutes ductus deferens, testicular and cremasteric arteries with the artery of ductus deferens, pampiniform plexus of veins, lymph vessels from testis, genital branch of genitofemoral nerve, and plexus of sympathetic nerves.

- *Coverings of Spermatic Cord*: From within outwards: internal spermatic fascia, cremasteric fascia, and external spermatic fascia.

Internal genital organs include:

Ductus or Vas Deferens

- Thick-walled, 45 cm long muscular tube transports spermatozoa from the epididymis to the ejaculatory duct. It has a narrow lumen except in the terminal part called the ampulla.

- Branches of superior, middle, and inferior vesical artery.

- Drains into the internal iliac veins.

- Parasympathetic fibers from the pelvic splanchnic nerves.

Seminal Vesicles

- Pyramidal (5 * 3 cm) organs between the urinary bladder's base and the rectum's ampulla.

- The duct of the seminal vesicle joins the ductus deferens to form the ejaculatory duct. Their secretions form a large amount of seminal fluid.

- Inferior vesical and middle rectal arteries.

- Sympathetic nerves from the superior hypogastric plexus and parasympathetic fibers from pelvic splanchnic nerves.

Ejaculatory Ducts

- Each duct is about 2 cm long and is formed by a union of vas deferens and duct of the seminal vesicle at the base of the prostate gland. The duct opens into the prostatic part of the urethra below and on each side of the prostatic utricle.

Prostate

- Pyramidal-shaped, fibromuscular glandular organ that surrounds the prostatic urethra. In females, the prostate is represented by the paraurethral glands (of Skene). Its secretions form the bulk of the seminal fluid.

- It resembles an inverted cone, measuring about 4 cm transversely at the base, 3 cm in length, and 2 cm in thickness. It weighs about 8 g.

- *The Prostate is Divided into Five Lobes*: anterior lobe (isthmus, devoid of glandular tissue), posterior lobe (site of carcinoma), median lobe (site of adenoma), and two lateral lobes (adenoma).

- Branches of the inferior vesical, middle rectal, and internal pudendal arteries.

- The venous drainage of the prostate follows two pathways:

1. Prostatic venous plexus → internal iliac veins → IVC. (Spread of metastasis of cancer prostate into the heart and lungs).

2. Prostatic venous plexus → vertebral venous plexus (of Batson) → intracranial dural venous sinuses (Spread of metastasis of cancer prostate into the vertebral column and brain).

■ Internal iliac, external iliac, and sacral groups of the lymph nodes.

■ Sympathetic supply is by the superior hypogastric plexus, and parasympathetic supply is by the pelvic splanchnic nerves.

PATHOLOGY

Case 126 OSVIRA (Zinner's Syndrome)

An 80-year-old male patient presented with abdominal pain and distension (Figure 6.2).

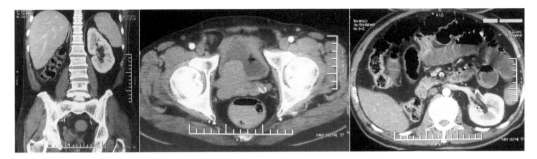

Figure 6.2 CECT abdomen depicts moderately dilated jejunal loops without signs of bowel infarction, perforation, or transition point. Partial thrombus (arrows) is seen in the proximal superior mesenteric artery apart from the absent right kidney and non-enhancing hypodense lesion in the region of the right seminal vesicle.

Discussion

Both ureteral buds and seminal vesicles develop from the mesonephric (Wolfian) duct; congenital seminal vesicle abnormalities are frequently associated with the ipsilateral upper urinary system. A first-trimester insult harms the kidney, ureter, seminal vesicle, and vas deferens development. Zinner's syndrome constitutes the triad of unilateral renal agenesis, ipsilateral seminal vesicle cyst, and ejaculatory duct obstruction. OSVIRA (Obstructed Seminal Vesicles with Ipsilateral Renal Agenesis) is also considered the male version of the female disorder—OHVIRA discussed in Chapter 5.

Patients may present with perineal pain, painful ejection, or infertility or may be detected incidentally, as in this case.

CT allows for the precise delineation of the renal and pelvic system abnormalities. The ipsilateral seminal vesicle, lying superior to the prostate gland, is enlarged along with fluid density and thin wall or hyperdense contents in the seminal vesicle cyst. MRI is superior due to its excellent soft tissue resolution, multiplanar capability, and nonionizing nature and shows a low signal on T1WI and high on T2WI.

This patient presented with acute abdominal pain and distension due to intestinal obstruction secondary to partial SMA thrombosis, which signifies that radiologists should not be biased by history and satisfaction of search. Mesenteric ischemia is discussed in Chapter 8.

Management

Surgery for symptomatic patients and conservative approach for asymptomatic patients.

Case 127 Benign Prostatic Hyperplasia

A 58-year-old male with urinary hesitancy (Figure 6.3).

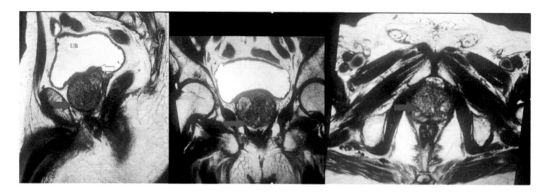

Figure 6.3 MRI pelvis depicts an enlarged prostate with a volume of 51 g—multiple scattered heterogeneous nodules with cystic areas in the transition zone surrounded by a hypointense capsule. Median lobar hypertrophy causing indentation of the bladder base. Mild irregularly thickened bladder wall.

Discussion

Benign prostatic hyperplasia (BPH) frequently affects men after the 5th–6th decade of life and presents with frequent nocturnal micturition, urinary retention, weak urinary stream, and incomplete bladder emptying. Untreated BPH may present as frequent urinary infections, urinary retention, calculus disease, and eventually renal failure. The prostate gland comprises three glandular zones: peripheral, transitional, and central zones and a stromal zone. BPH causes enlargement involving the transitional and stromal zone and the sub-sphincteric peri-urethral region.

Sonography, the initial modality of choice, shows an enlarged central gland with a volume of more than 40 g apart from well-defined hypo/iso/hyperechoic nodules in the transition zone. Increased post-void residual volume, thickened and trabeculated urinary bladder wall with diverticula, and urinary system calculi are commonly encountered findings. Transrectal ultrasonography (TRUS)/MRI depicts various types of prostatic enlargements—bilateral TZ enlargement (corresponding to bilateral lobes of the prostate), retrourethral enlargement (deep peri urethral glands), and pedunculated enlargement (protruding prostatic nodules). Intravenous Urography and Retrograde Urography may show indentation on the elevated urinary bladder, resulting in lower ureteric deformity (J-hook, fish hook, or hockey stick).

Differential Diagnosis

Carcinoma prostate (nodules in the peripheral zone showing restricted diffusion).

Management

- Minimally invasive procedure such as trans-urethral resection of the prostate (TURP)
- Simple prostatectomy, laser ablation, or arterial embolization. However, laser ablations can distort the normal anatomy of the prostate. Strictures or abscesses may be seen in patients who undergo treatment for BPH.

Case 128 Prostate Carcinoma

A 72-year-old male with urinary retention (Figure 6.4).

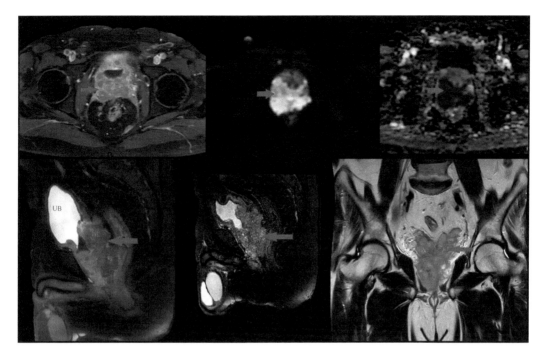

Figure 6.4 MRI pelvis reveals an enlarged prostate with heterogeneously enhancing, ill-defined, multilobulated T2 isointense lesion with the loss of normal T2 hyperintensity and restricted diffusion on DWI. The lesion breaches the capsule and infiltrates periprostatic fat, adjacent neurovascular bundles, muscular planes, the base of the urinary bladder (irregularly thickened bladder wall), bilateral seminal vesicles, rectum, and external anal sphincter.

Discussion

Prostate cancer, frequently the adenocarcinoma subtype, is a slow-growing disease that usually presents with urinary retention, hesitancy, and increased frequency (Figure 6.4). Patients may present with hematuria and backache as the disease spreads. The hard nodule is palpable on digital examination, and PSA (prostate-specific antigen) > 10 ng/mL mandates biopsy. Tumor spread is via

- Local infiltration into the bladder and urethra
- Lymphatic spread to inguinal and para-aortic nodes
- Hematogeneous spread to bones, lungs, etc.

Prostate carcinoma is frequent in the peripheral zone containing maximum glandular tissue. It may also be seen in central/transitional zones but not in the anterior fibromuscular stroma because of the absence of glandular tissue.

Transrectal Ultrasound (TRUS) shows a hypoechoic nodule with high vascularity, asymmetric bulge, and gland distortion in the PZ. However, TRUS does not differentiate between benign and malignant etiologies but helps guide biopsy or plan treatment. Multiparametric MRI (mp-MRI) includes morphological assessment by high-resolution T2WI along with any two functional MRI techniques (DWI, perfusion techniques, dynamic contrast scans, or spectroscopy). MRI is useful in determining extracapsular extension, radiotherapy response, and recurrence after radiotherapy—T2 hypointense nodule in the PZ, which is usually homogenously hyperintense. Malignant nodules often show restricted diffusion on DWI with an increased Choline: Citrate ratio on spectroscopy.

Pitfalls

- All hypoechoic/hypervascular nodules are not malignant, with about half being due to benign causes such as cysts, vessels, prostatitis, or glandular ectasias.
- 8–10-week wait between prostate biopsy and MRI examination is recommended.

Differentials

- Biopsy-related hemorrhage
- Changes from hormone therapy
- Prostatitis
- Postradiation fibrosis

Management

Prostatectomy and radiation therapy, including brachytherapy, HIFU, and cryotherapy, may all be used depending on the stage and extent of the disease.

Case 129 Testicular Malignancy with Pulmonary Metastasis

A 52-year-old male with a palpable mass in the right scrotum (Figure 6.5).

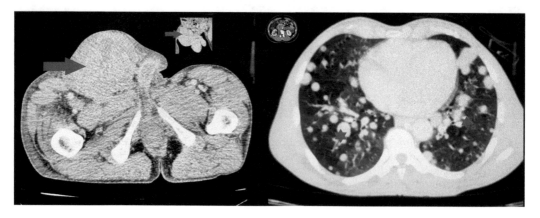

Figure 6.5 CECT abdomen depicts heterogeneously enhancing mass in the right scrotal sac with a few calcific foci and bulky right spermatic cord. Heterogeneous necrotic nodes were noted in the inguinal and retroperitoneal region, along with pulmonary cannonball metastasis.

Discussion

Testicular malignancy is common in young males, the risk factors being cryptorchidism, family history, and infertility. Germ cell tumors are the most frequent malignant types with seminomas and nonseminomatous (yolk sac carcinoma, embryonal carcinoma, choriocarcinoma, and teratoma) tumors. Sex-cord and stromal tumors are usually benign, the common ones being Sertoli-cell tumor, Leydig cell tumor, granulosa cell tumor, fibroma, thecoma, etc. Serum tumor markers, such as alpha-fetoprotein (AFP), beta human chorionic gonadotropin (β-hCG), and lactate dehydrogenase (LDH), are most commonly assessed in testicular malignancies. Seminoma is the most common type, with a propensity to involve retroperitoneal lymph nodes (first to involve) due to venous and lymphatic drainage. Later, it spreads to supraclavicular nodes and distant organs. Imaging reveals solid, well-defined hypoechoic/attenuated intratesticular lesions with heterogeneous enhancement.

Table 6.1 depicts the staging of testicular tumor.

Table 6.1: **Staging of Testicular Tumor**

Stage		Distant Metastasis	Nodal Involvement
Stage 1	T1: Testis, epididymis T2: Extension to tunica albuginea/vaginalis T3: Invades spermatic cord T4: Invades scrotum	No	No
Stage 2	T1: T4	No	Retroperitoneal spread
Stage 3	T1: T4	Yes (pulmonary, liver, and bones)	Yes

Differential Diagnosis

- Infarct
- Infection
- Trauma

Management

- Orchiectomy with chemoradiotherapy.
- Seminoma is radiosensitive tumor.

Case 130 Penile Carcinoma

A 59-year-old male with irregular lump on penis (Figure 6.6).

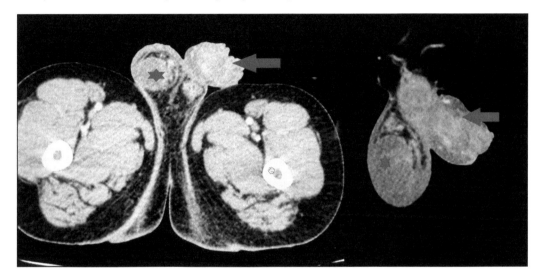

Figure 6.6 Ill-defined irregularly marginated heterogeneously enhancing with a few non-enhancing necrotic areas involving the glans penis infiltrating both corpora cavernosa and corpora spongiosum with skin irregularities. Mild bilateral hydrocele.

Discussion

Primary penile malignancy, usually squamous cell carcinoma, is infrequent and affects elderly males, the glans and foreskin being the most common locations. The common risk factors are poor hygiene, sexually transmitted infections, obesity, smoking, ultraviolet rays, etc. though circumcision is considered protective. Eryhthroplasia of Queyrat and Bowen's disease are premalignant lesions. Patients present with irregular lump, foul-smelling discharge, pain, and itching. CT/MRI/PET scan delineates the extent of the lesion and lymphadenopathy, assesses the staging, and helps plan treatment.

Differentials

Metastasis, lymphoma, etc.

Management

Surgery

Case 131 Cryptorchidism

A 13-year-old male wih empty left scrotal sac (Figure 6.7).

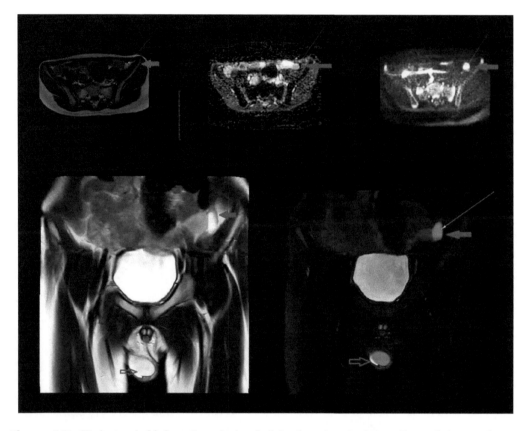

Figure 6.7 Undescended left testis at the level of the deep inguinal ring. Empty left scrotal sac. A well-defined oval T1 isointense, T2/STIR hyperintense structure showing restricted diffusion on DWI was noted in the left inguinal canal at the level of the deep inguinal ring—undescended left testis. Normal right testis in the right scrotal sac.

Discussion

Generally, the testis develops intra-abdominally and relocates to the scrotum by up to 30 weeks through the inguinal canal. Risk factors a/w cryptorchidism include prematurity, gestational diabetes, and syndromes like Prader-Willi, etc., with a high propensity for infertility, torsion, and testicular malignancy if not operated on.

Sonography reveals a homogeneously hypoechoic oval structure with echogenic mediastinum testis high up in the inguinal canal or anywhere along the course of its descent. Empty ipsilateral scrotal sac and normal contralateral sac. MRI is better at identifying the undescended testis.

Differential

Retractile testis- freely mobile, fully descended testis that changes position due to hyperactive cremasteric reflex. Descends at puberty without increased risk for infertility.

Management

If the testis remains undescended, ideally by 6 months, orchiopexy should be performed.

SUGGESTED READINGS

Drake, R. L., & Vogl, A. W. (2020). *Gray's Atlas of Anatomy E-Book*. Elsevier Health Science.

Lumley, J. S., & Craven, J. L. (2018). *Bailey & Love's Essential Clinical Anatomy*. CRC Press.

Mittal, P. K. et al. Role of imaging in the evaluation of male infertility. *Radiographics* 2017;37:3, 837–854.

7 Aorta and IVC

EMBRYOLOGY

The twin dorsal aortae fuse during fetal development to form the abdominal aorta. The six aortic arches/pharyngeal arch arteries originating from the aortic sac in the fetal head are continuous with the paired dorsal aortae. These six pairs of embryologic vascular structures develop into the great arteries of the head and neck, including parts of the common carotid artery, internal carotid artery, maxillary artery, aortic arch, pulmonary artery, right subclavian artery, ductus arteriosus, stapedial artery, and hyoid artery.

ANATOMY

The thoracic aorta is divided into three parts: the ascending aorta, the aortic arch, and the descending aorta. The ascending part originates via the left ventricle anterior to the pulmonary artery and reaches superiorly up to the T4 vertebrae level. The second division, which arches posteriorly and to the left, is known as the arch of the aorta, giving off three branches, namely the brachiocephalic trunk (innominate artery), left common carotid artery, and left subclavian artery, and continues as descending thoracic aorta from T4 vertebral level until it reaches diaphragm. The retroperitoneal abdominal aorta enters the abdomen via the aortic hiatus caudal to the xiphoid process. It rests anterior to the vertebral body and parallel to the inferior vena cava. Extending about 1– cm below the umbilicus, the aorta divides into the common iliac arteries at the level of L4. The aorta diminishes in size as it descends through the abdominal cavity, moving more superficially as well. After exiting the diaphragm into the abdomen, posterior to median arcuate ligament, the abdominal aorta (AA) gives rise to paired (inferior phrenic, mid adrenal, renal, and gonadal) and unpaired (celiac, SMA, IMA, and median sacral) arteries and subsequently bifurcates into the common iliac arteries at L4 vertebrae level. AA descends anteriorly and to the left of the lumbar vertebrae with IVC on its right side.

Extensive arterial collaterals develop to compensate for AA blockage.

Radiologists should consider any anatomical variations of the AA before using diagnostic imaging techniques like angiography and therapeutic interventions or surgeries.

Crucial Anastomosis

- Superior pancreaticoduodenal branch of celiac artery with inferior pancreaticoduodenal branch of SMA at duodenum.

- Middle colic branch of SMA and inferior colic branch of IMA at distal transverse colon.

- Superior rectal branch of IMA and inferior rectal branch of the internal iliac artery at the rectum.

The marginal artery of Drummond forms anastomosis between the terminal branches of SMA and IMA, extending from the ileocecal junction to the rectosigmoid junction, though it is poorly developed in watershed areas of splenic flexure and rectosigmoid region, making them prone to ischemia.

Branches of the AA in descending order are discussed (Table 7.1 and Figure 7.1).

Table 7.1: Branches of abdominal aorta

Artery	Number	Origin	Supply
Inferior phrenic	Paired	Posteriorly at T12 level	Diaphragm
Celiac (branches into left gastric, common hepatic, and splenic arteries)	Unpaired	Anteriorly at the level of T12	Foregut (Liver, spleen, stomach, proximal duodenum, and pancreas)
SMA (branches into superior pancreaticoduodenal, middle, right, and ileocolic arteries)	Unpaired	Anteriorly, at lower L1	Midgut (distal duodenum, jejunum, ileum, ascending colon, and proximal transverse colon)
Middle suprarenal	Paired	Posteriorly at L1	Adrenal glands

(Continued)

DOI: 10.1201/9781003452034-7

Table 7.1: (*Continued*) Branches of abdominal aorta

Artery	Number	Origin	Supply
Renal	Paired	Laterally between L1 and L2	Kidneys
Gonadal	Paired	Laterally, at L2 level	Testes/ovaries
IMA (branches into left colic, sigmoid, and superior rectal arteries)	Unpaired	Anteriorly at L3	Hindgut (from splenic flexure to proximal rectum)
Median sacral	Unpaired	Posteriorly at L4	Coccyx, lumbar vertebrae, and sacrum
Lumbar	Four pairs	Posterolaterally between L1–4	Abdominal wall, spinal cord
Common iliac	Paired	Bifurcation at L4	Lower limb, pelvic viscera, and gluteal region

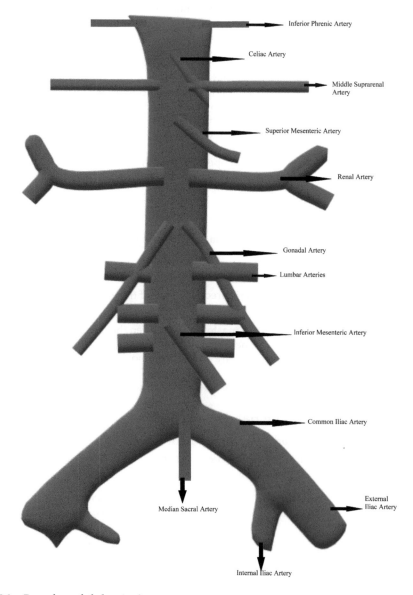

Figure 7.1 Branches of abdominal aorta.

DEVELOPMENT OF IVC

Embryology

Embryological venous systems

1. Vitelline system (drains GIT)

2. Umbilical system (drains placenta)

3. Cardinal system (rest of body)

Development of normal IVC

1. Hepatic IVC (right vitelline vein)

2. Infrahepatic IVC

    • Suprarenal IVC (right subcardinal vein)

    • Renal IVC (supracardinal and subcardinal veins anastomosis)

    • Infrarenal IVC (posterior cardinal veins)

Anatomy

The inferior vena cava (IVC) is formed by the confluence of the right and left common iliac veins at the L5 vertebral level and lies toward the right side of the vertebral column. It enters the heart's right atrium after passing through the diaphragm at the T8 level. Blood from the abdominal viscera travels into the portal vein and enters the IVC via the hepatic veins after traversing the liver and its sinusoids.

Various tributaries of IVC (Table 7.2)

Table 7.2: Tributaries of IVC

Lumbar veins	L1–5
Right gonadal vein	L2
Renal veins	L1
Right suprarenal vein	L1
Hepatic veins	T8
Inferior phrenic veins	T8

The left gonadal and suprarenal veins drain into the left renal vein.

Normal Variant

Pseudolipoma of IVC

Partial volume artifact due to a layer of fat that lies above the caudate lobe next to the IVC simulates fatty mass in the lumen of the inferior vena cava. It gets more prominent in cirrhosis due to shrunken liver and anatomic distortion. It should be differentiated from true lipoma and vascular thrombus.

IVC Variants

Duplex IVC, left-sided IVC, absent infrarenal IVC with azygous continuation, and retro-aortic/circum-aortic left renal vein.

Retro-aortic left renal vein (Figure 7.2)

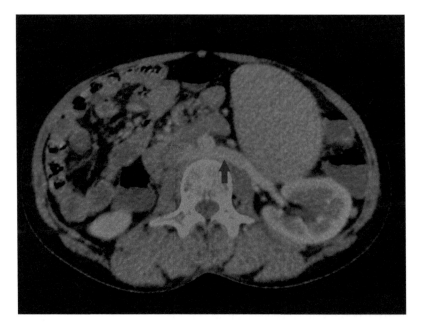

Figure 7.2 Left renal vein (arrow) passes posterior to the aorta (A) before draining to IVC.

Circum-aortic left renal vein (Figure 7.3)

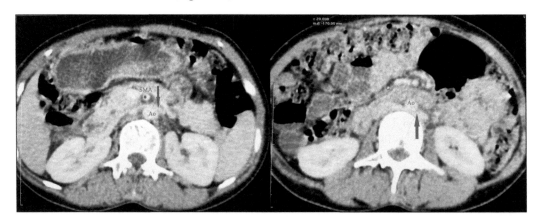

Figure 7.3 The left renal vein passes anterior (between SMA and aorta) and posterior (between aorta and vertebral body) to the aorta.

Case 132 Duplex IVC

Discussion

An incidental note was made of the clinically insignificant anomaly of isolated duplicated IVC due to a persistent left supracardinal vein that joins anterior to the renal arteries to form suprarenal IVC (Figure 7.4). It is important in renal transplant cases.

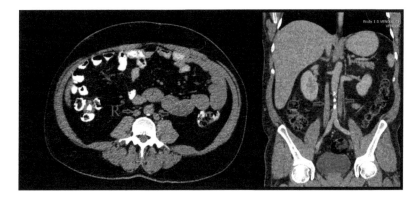

Figure 7.4 Three-vessel pattern with aorta sandwiched between right and left IVC (open arrows).

Differential Diagnosis

1. Lymph node

2. Left pyeloureteric dilatation

3. Left-sided IVC (transposition of IVC)

Case 133 Aortic Aneurysm

A 77-year-old male smoker (Figure 7.5).

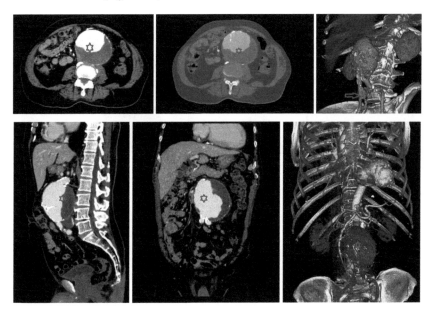

Figure 7.5 CECT abdomen. Long segment aneurysmal dilatation (10.3*9.5*8.9 of infrarenal abdominal aorta approximately 4.5 cm distal to the origin of renal arteries extending till its bifurcation with no extension into iliac vessels. Peripheral calcified atheromatous plaques and a calcified membrane are seen within the non-thrombosed portion of the aneurysm arising from the anterior wall. No apparent features of aortic dissection are seen. Another small fusiform non-thrombosed aneurysm (red arrow) in the right common iliac artery extends to its bifurcation.

Discussion

AAA are focal dilatations>3 cm. It may be fusiform (circumferential expansion) or saccular (localized outpouchings), the most common location being infrarenal, and the most common cause is atherosclerosis (Figure 7.5). They are common in elderly males, smokers, whites, and hypertensives. Patients are usually asymptomatic but may present as pulsatile mass with abdominal or back pain. Sonography is ideally used for screening and monitoring unruptured aneurysms. Helical CT and CTA produce 3D images of the aneurysm, determining its size, anatomy, and relation to critical adjacent structures. NCCT. Thrombus should be included to measure the diameter accurately. Intimal flaps, if present, suggest aortic dissection.

Complications include rupture resulting in retroperitoneal hemorrhage, contrast extravasation, adjacent fat stranding, and hypotensive shock. The other complications are pseudoaneurysm, distal thromboembolism, aortocaval and aortoenteric fistulas.

Management

- Surgery is recommended if the size is >5 cm or rapid increase in size on serial monitoring.

- Endovascular stent-grafts.

Case 134 Embolized Gastroduodenal Artery Pseudoaneurysm

A 42-year-old male presented with abdominal pain and a known history of pancreatitis and melaena (Figure 7.6).

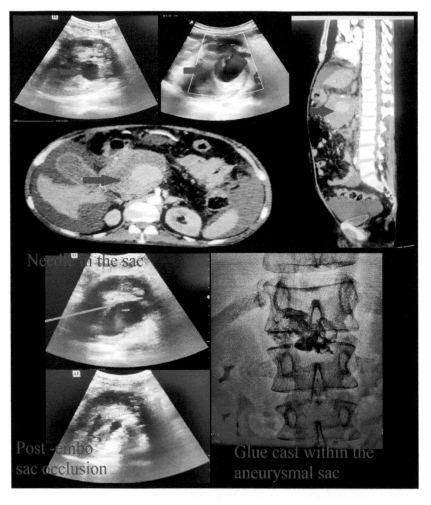

Figure 7.6 Sonography shows an anechoic lesion surrounded by echogenic thrombosis. CDUS shows turbulent arterial blood flow with a bidirectional flow pattern and yin-yang sign. CECT abdomen depicts a homogeneously enhancing GDA aneurysm in the pancreatic head region surrounded by a non-enhancing thrombus. Percutaneous direct puncture technique was used to embolize using vividol and glue.

Discussion

Gastroduodenal artery (GDA) aneurysms are infrequent visceral artery aneurysms, the common sites being the hepatic and splenic arteries. Unruptured aneurysms remain clinically silent, but ruptured aneurysms may be fatal and present with shock and hemodynamic instability. The main etiological factors in the formation of GDA aneurysms include:

■ Traumatic/inflammatory vascular injuries, mainly pancreatitis (disruption of the vessel wall due to pancreatic enzyme leakage in patients), and vascular/surgical interventions for false aneurysms

■ Vessel wall abnormalities/atherosclerosis (weakening of arterial wall) for true aneurysms.

CT scan better determines the vascular anatomy, aneurysm origin, and extent, preparing better for surgical repair. Angiography is the gold standard modality that is both diagnostic and therapeutic.

Management

■ *Asymptomatic*: Should be treated due to its propensity to rupture. Planned endovascular approach, including ultrasound-guided thrombin injection, embolization, or stent grafting.

■ *Ruptured*: Depending on the hemodynamic stability of the patient.

• Endovascular approach

• Emergency laparotomy

Case 135 Superior Mesenteric Artery Syndrome/Wilkie Syndrome
A 16-year-old asthenic female with abdominal distension and vomiting (Figure 7.7).

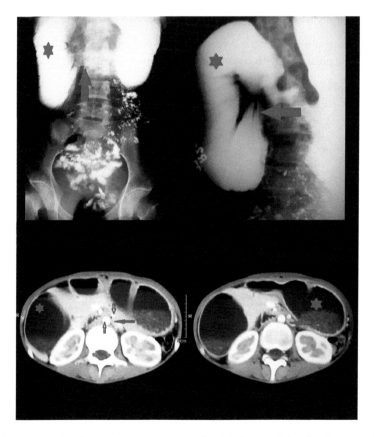

Figure 7.7 Barium study shows abrupt cut-off at the third part of the duodenum with persistent contrast pooling in the proximal part. CECT abdomen depicts compression of the third part of the duodenum with upstream dilatation.

Discussion

Superior mesenteric artery (SMA) syndrome, an aortomesenteric duodenal compression syndrome, is a rare vascular compression syndrome where the third part of the duodenum gets compressed between the aorta and SMA, resulting in dilatation of the proximal duodenum and stomach. It may be congenital (shortened ligament of Treitz), or a/w prolonged bed rest in a supine position (body cast) prior to scoliosis surgery (relative lengthening of the spine with SMA displacement superiorly altering the aortomesenteric angle), exaggerated lumbar lordosis.

It is frequent in young asthenic females with weight loss (loss of mesenteric fat cushioning around the duodenum) and presents with progressive postprandial vomiting, abdominal fullness, etc., and the symptoms improve in the prone/knee-elbow position/left lateral decubitus position.

Barium studies reveal abrupt termination due to extrinsic compression of the third part of the duodenum with proximal dilatation and distal collapse of bowel loops. Normal aortomesenteric angle and aorto mesenteric distance are 28°–64° and 10–32 mm, better delineated on CTA and MRA images, which get reduced to <20° and <8 mm, respectively.

Differentials of Dilated Stomach and duodenum

- Aganglionosis
- Scleroderma
- Diabetic gastroparesis

Management

- Conservative approach with initial NGT decompression, nutritional rehabilitation, and positioning maneuvers.
- Duodenojejunostomy (endoscopic/surgical) in complicated cases.

Case 136 Mesenteric Arterial Steal Syndrome (Arc of Riolan)

A 37-year-old female presented with chronic abdominal pain (Figure 7.8).

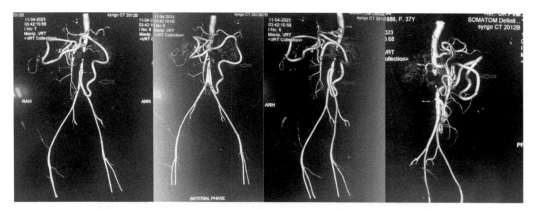

Figure 7.8   Abdominal angiographic reconstructed images show mesenteric steal with retrograde flow via an Arc of Riolan to perfuse aortoiliac circulation. Depicts a complete block (solid red arrow) in the infrarenal portion of the abdominal aorta with the paucity of mesenteric vessels. Prominent abnormal tortuous artery (expansion of Arc of Riolan—open red arrow) providing collateral flow is noted.

Discussion

Arc of Riolan, an arterio-arterial anastomosis that usually develops in chronic atherosclerotic occlusion, as a collateral channel linking proximal SMA or its main branches to proximal IMA or its main branches. It is tortuous and prominent, runs close to the mesenteric root (medially), and is also known as a central anastomotic mesenteric artery, meandering mesenteric artery, and is diagnostic of SMA/IMA occlusion. Extensive collaterals between splanchnic vessels form a protective mechanism against ischemia.

Differentials

Marginal artery of Drummond lies in the peripheral mesentery of the colon.
   Arc of Buhler—embryologic remnant between celiac trunk and SMA.
   Arc of Barkow—anastomotic channel between right (GDA) and left (splenic artery) gastroepi-
ploic arteries.

Management

Endovascular revascularization with balloon-expandable stent
   Surgery

Case 137 SMV Thrombosis

A 54-year-old female with acute abdominal pain (Figure 7.9).

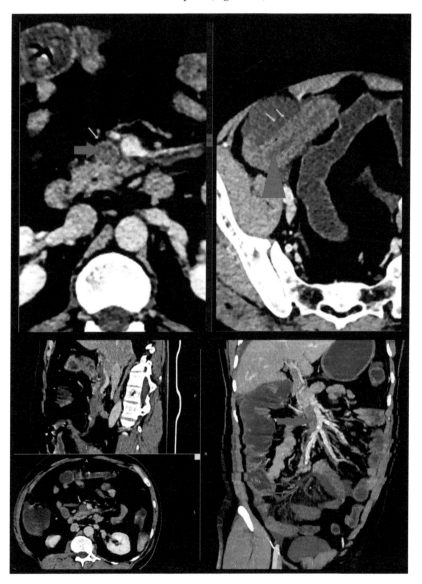

Figure 7.9 CECT abdomen depicts occlusive thrombus (solid arrow) in SMV, its ileal tributaries, portal vein confluence, and right branch of the portal vein. Long segment of ileum with circumferential edematous hypodense hypoenhancing wall thickening in distal ileal loops (arrowhead) s/o ischemic bowel. Dilated ileal veins along the vasa recta give a comb sign with mesenteric fat stranding and mild ascites.

Discussion

SMV thrombosis can be acute/chronic or primary (idiopathic)/secondary (hypercoagulable states, pancreatitis, pancreatic neoplasms, mesenteric venous stasis—Budd Chiari syndrome, recent surgery, etc).

Acute cases present with colicky abdominal pain and haem-positive stools.

CT reveals

- Filling defects in SMV or its branches

- Thickened edematous (hypoattenuating)/hemorrhagic (hyperattenuating) bowel wall with indistinct margins and abnormal enhancement

- Luminal distension

- Ascites

- Mesenteric congestion and fat stranding

Blockage of venous drainage increases hydrostatic pressure, fluid accumulation, and a layered pattern of enhancement due to hyperdensity in mucosa and submucosa due to increased flow. Arterial obstruction raises intestinal wall tension, leading to hypodensity due to infarction.

Collaterals develop in chronic mesenteric venous thrombosis, averts infarction but leads to bleeding due to venous hypertension.

Differentials

Acute mesenteric ischemia can be arterial/venous/non-occlusive/strangulating bowel obstruction types.

- *NOMI (Non-Occlusive Mesenteric Ischemia)*: Low output state with extensive pneumatosis, small caliber aorta, collapsed IVC, and hyper-enhancing adrenals.

- Strangulating bowel obstruction is noted in closed-loop obstruction with decreased bowel wall enhancement and hazy mesentery.

Management

Surgery or endovascular treatment, depending on the etiology.

Case 138 Nutcracker Syndrome

An 18-year-old male with flank pain (Figure 7.10).

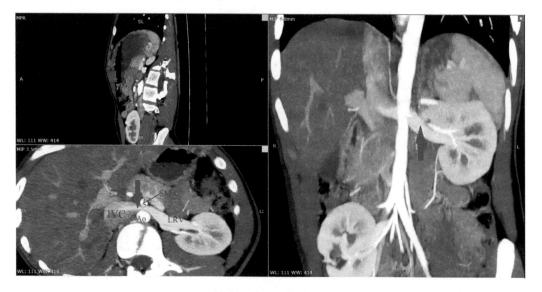

Figure 7.10 CT abdomen depicting entrapped LRV (solid arrow) between the aorta and SMA (star).

Discussion

Nutcracker phenomenon, the LRV entrapment between the aorta and SMA, is usually asymptomatic. In comparison, nutcracker syndrome results in hematuria and flank pain due to LRV compression, leading to high pressure and resultant collateral formation. It may also result in varices at the hilum, causing varicocele (infertility) in males and ovarian vein syndrome/pelvic congestion syndrome in females.

Differentials

Circum-aortic LRV constitutes a duplicated LRV with pre-aortic (anterior) and retro-aortic (posterior) components forming a cuff around the AA.

Management

LRV stenting/transposition considering age and severity of disease.

Case 139 Renal Artery Stenting

A 20-year-old patient with refractory hypertension (Figure 7.11).

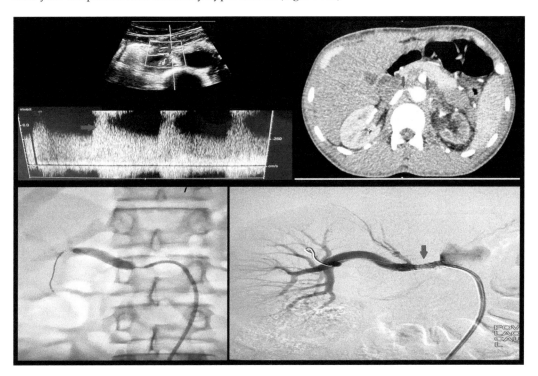

Figure 7.11 Sonography, doppler (parvus tardus flow), and CECT reveals right renal artery stenosis >90% and non-visualized left renal artery with collaterals—critical stenosis treated with angioplasty and stenting.

Discussion

Patients with worsening renal function and malignant hypertension resistant to antihypertensive medications are treated with interventional techniques to restore blood flow within stenosed renal arteries due to atherosclerosis or fibromuscular dysplasia. Percutaneous transluminal renal angioplasty is better for non-ostial lesions and lesions with <50% stenosis, and stenting is better for the lesions at the ostium causing refractory hypertension and >60%–70% renal artery stenosis. Complications include vessel injury, embolization, or site hematoma.

Points to Note

- In cases of bilateral RAS, a procedure should be attempted to treat both vessels simultaneously.

- Stent should include the aortic part to ostium to a few mm distal to the stenosis.

- Gap within stents may cause intimal hyperplasia, though overlapping stents decrease patency.

- A repeat angiogram is required to assess stenosis or abnormal pressure gradients.

SUGGESTED READINGS

Litmanovich, D. CT and MRI in diseases of the aorta. *Am J Roentgenol.* 2009;193(4):928–940. doi: 10.2214/AJR.08.2166.

Smillie, R. P., Shetty, M., Boyer, A. C. et al. Imaging evaluation of the inferior vena cava. *Radiographics.* 2015;35:2, 578–592.

8 Diaphragm, Peritoneum, Retroperitoneum, and Anterior Abdominal Wall

EMBRYOLOGY AND ANATOMY

Diaphragm

The diaphragm is a musculotendinous sheath that divides the pleuropericardial (thoracic cavity) and peritoneal (abdominal cavity) membranes.

The diaphragm develops during 4–12 weeks of embryogenesis and arises from four major components:

- Transverse septum (forms the central tendon of the diaphragm)

- Pleuroperitoneal folds

- Dorsal mesentery of the esophagus

- Lateral body wall musculature

Pleuroperitoneal folds appear in the fifth week, fuse with septum transversum, and dorsal mesentery of the esophagus around the seventh week divides thoracic and abdominal cavities. The body wall forms the peripheral rim (Figure 8.1).

Origin

- Sternal part arises from the posterior part of the xiphoid process.

- Costal part arises from the deep surfaces of the last six ribs and their coastal cartilages.

- Vertebral part originates from vertical columns and the arcuate ligaments.

- Right crus arises from the sides of the first three vertebral bodies and intervening cartilages.

- Left crus arises from the sides of the first two vertebral bodies and intervening cartilages.

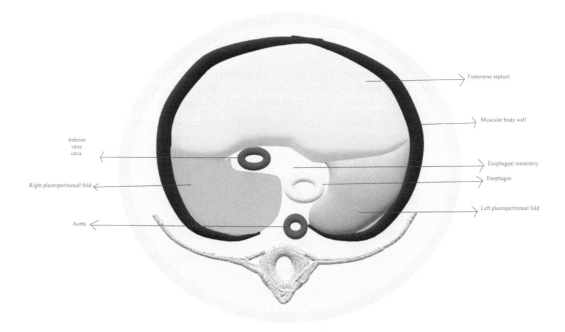

Figure 8.1 Major components of the diaphragm.

DOI: 10.1201/9781003452034-8

- Medial arcuate ligament arches from the lateral side of the body of L2 and reaches up to the transverse process tip of L1 bilaterally.

- Lateral arcuate ligament arches from the transverse process of the L1 vertebral body to the inferior border of the 12th rib.

- Median arcuate ligament is formed by a connection between two cruras that cover the aorta.

Insertion—the diaphragm is seen inserting into the central tendon.
Openings in the diaphragm (Table 8.1)

Table 8.1: Diaphragmatic openings

Opening	Level	Structures Traversing through the Opening
Caval	T8	IVC, right phrenic nerve
Esophageal	T10	Esophagus, bilateral vagus nerves, esophageal branches from left gastric vessels, lymphatics, sympathetic nerves
Aortic	T12	Aorta, azygous vein, thoracic duct

Other openings include sympathetic splanchnic nerves that pierce the crura, the sympathetic plexus that passes posterior to the medial arcuate ligament on both sides and the superior epigastric vessels that pass between the sternal and costal origin of the esophagus on both sides.

Peritoneum

The embryonic lateral plate mesoderm cleaves to form somatic (parietal) and splanchnic (visceral) layers of the peritoneum. Primitive gut tube and peritoneum develop simultaneously during embryonic life, suggesting the continuity of spaces within. The developing primitive gut tube is anchored by the ventral and dorsal mesenteries of the peritoneum to the anterior and posterior abdominal wall. These mesenteries contain blood vessels to supply the primitive gut.

The abdominal (celomic) cavity extends from the diaphragm to the pelvic floor and is divided into the peritoneal and extraperitoneal compartments. The peritoneum is a continuous serous membrane covering the abdominal viscera. The superficial parietal and deep visceral layers, separated by approximately 50 ml serous fluid, enclose the peritoneal cavity.

Peritoneal folds connect organs or to the anterior and posterior abdominal wall through mesentery, ligaments, and omentum.

- Mesentery is a double fold of visceral peritoneum. The mesentery of the small intestine, meso-appendix, transverse mesocolon, and sigmoid mesocolon connect the jejuno-ileum, appendix, transverse colon, and sigmoid colon to the posterior abdominal wall, respectively.

- Ligaments are two layers of peritoneum that are named by connecting parts such as gastrosplenic, gastro phrenic, gastrocolic, hepatogastric (stomach and spleen, diaphragm, transverse colon, and liver), phrenicocolic (diaphragm and transverse colon), splenorenal (spleen and kidneys), hepatoduodenal (portahepatis of liver and duodenum; contains portal triad) and falciform ligament (liver and anterior abdominal wall).

- Omenta are layered sheets of the peritoneum (Table 8.2).

Table 8.2: Types of Omenta

Greater Omentum	Lesser Omentum
Four-layered peritoneal fold	Two-layered fold
Extends from the greater curvature of the stomach and covers the transverse colon and intestines	Covers lesser curvature of the stomach, duodenum, and liver
Includes gastrosplenic, gastrophrenic, and gastrocolic ligaments	Includes hepatogastric and hepatoduodenal ligaments
Component of dorsal mesentery	Ventral mesentery

Classification depending on peritoneal covering (Table 8.3).

Table 8.3: **Classification of Organs Depending on Peritoneal Covering**

Intraperitoneal	Retroperitoneal
Organs fully covered by visceral peritoneum	Organs located behind the posterior parietal peritoneum
Liver, spleen, stomach, duodenum (first part), pancreatic tail, jejunum, ileum, appendix, transverse and sigmoid colon, upper one-third rectum, uterus fundus and body, ovaries	Rest of duodenum and pancreas, IVC, aorta kidneys, adrenals, proximal ureters, ascending and descending colon, and middle one-third rectum, anal canal
Structures are usually mobile	Relatively fixed
Connected by mesentery	Not connected by mesentery

Lower one-third of rectum, distal ureter, urinary bladder, prostate, seminal vesicles, uterus, and fallopian tubes are subperitoneal.

The peritoneal cavity is divided into several spaces, primarily into greater and lesser sacs by omenta and transverse mesocolon (Table 8.4).

Table 8.4: **Division of Peritoneal Spaces (Greater Sac vs Lesser Sac)**

Greater Sac	Lesser Sac (Omental Bursa)
Anterior part of the cavity from diaphragm to pelvis	Posterosuperior part of the cavity
Subdivided into supracolic (liver, spleen, stomach) and infracolic (small intestine, ascending and descending colon) spaces by transverse mesocolon	Posterior to stomach and liver and anterior to pancreas and duodenum
Paracolic gutters help in free communication with greater sac compartments	Epiploic foramen on its free edge helps in communication with the greater sac

The subphrenic recess is the highest point, and the rectouterine/vesical pouch is the lowest point in the peritoneal cavity (Figure 8.2).

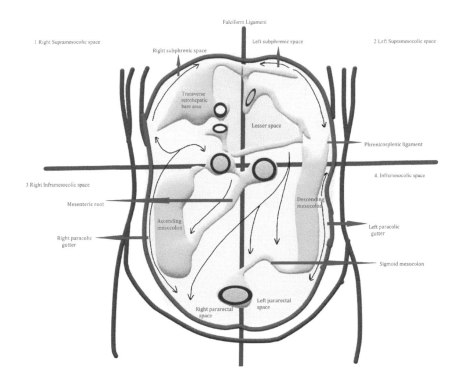

Figure 8.2 The peritoneal spaces.

Retroperitoneum

The retroperitoneum extends from the diaphragm to the pelvis and is situated between the posterior parietal peritoneum and transversalis fascia of the posterior abdominal wall. Organs that were initially attached to mesentery and later migrated retroperitoneally were called secondary retroperitoneal organs (duodenum, pancreas, and ascending and descending colon) compared to primary retroperitoneal organs that were retroperitoneal since the inception of development. It is divided into a few anatomic spaces (Table 8.5)

Table 8.5: Retroperitoneal Anatomic Spaces

Anterior Pararenal Space	Perirenal Space (Inverted Cone)	Posterior Pararenal Space	Great Vessel Space
Pancreas, duodenum, ascending and descending colon	Adrenal glands, kidney, renal vessels, ureters, lymph, and fat	Fat, vessels, lymphatics Bridging renorenal septa	Aorta, IVC, and fat
Posterior parietal peritoneum (posteriorly), anterior renal fascia (anteriorly)	Anterior (Gerotas's) and posterior (Zuckerandl) renal fascia	Posterior renal fascia (anteriorly) and transversalis fascia (posteriorly)	Anterior to vertebral bodies
Continuous across the midline	Do not communicate directly (Kneeland channel is a hypothetical connection between two spaces)	Communicates with contralateral space through preperitoneal space	Superiorly it is continuous with posterior mediastinum

The posterior compartment includes psoas muscles. Retroperitoneal space is compartmentalized into sub-spaces containing fat and loose connective tissue via interfascial planes. Multilaminated renal and lateroconal fascia include potential spaces, with retrorenal, retromesenteric, and lateroconal planes communicating at fascial trifurcation. This results in the interfascial spread of fluid collections and disease pathologies to other parts. Spaces may communicate to the pelvis by following the ureter. The pelvis may be compartmentalized into five spaces, namely, prevesical, paravesical, perivesical, presacral, and perirectal spaces (Figure 8.3).

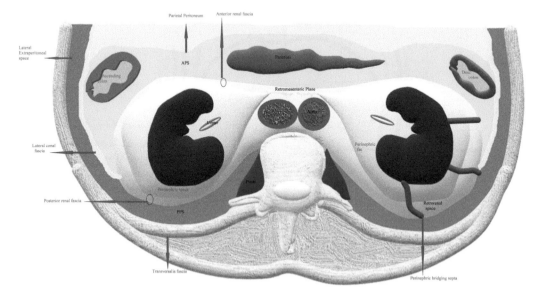

Figure 8.3 Anatomical spaces of the retroperitoneum.

Anterior Abdominal Wall

It is limited above by the xiphisternum and costal margins, below by the iliac crest and pubic bones, and laterally by the midaxillary line. The abdominal wall is primarily supplied by epigastric arteries and innervated by thoracoabdominal nerves.

Layers of Anterior Abdominal Wall

It has eight layers from before backward, reduced to six opposite linea alba.

1. The *skin* of the anterior abdominal wall is capable of stretching. Undue stretching causes white streaks known as lineae albicantes.

   Umbilicus: It is a normal scar on the anterior abdominal wall. It represents the fetal end of the umbilical cord. In healthy adults, it lies at the level of intervertebral discs between the third and fourth lumbar vertebrae. In newborns and old age, it lies at a lower level. It marks the watershed line of the body, with reference to venous and lymphatic drainage, and is an essential site of portocaval anastomosis. In portal hypertension, these anastomoses open to form dilated veins known as caput medusae.

2. *Superficial Fascia* is a layer of fatty connective tissue, a single layer up to the umbilicus, and below splits into a superficial fatty layer (Camper's fascia) and a deep membranous layer (Scarpa's fascia). The fascia contains cutaneous nerves, vessels, and lymphatics.

3. *External Oblique*

   Inguinal ligament: Lower-free border of external oblique aponeurosis, between anterior superior iliac spine and pubic tubercle.

   Superficial inguinal ring aponeurosis presents a triangular gap above the pubic symphysis.

4. *Internal Oblique*

   Lower aponeurotic fibers of internal oblique and transversus abdominis muscles fuse to form *Conjoint Tendon or Falx Inguinalis*, which arches over the spermatic cord and is attached to the pubic crest and pectineus.

5. *Transversus Abdominis*

   The neurovascular plane of the abdominal wall lies between the internal oblique and transversus abdominis muscle.

6. *Fascia Transversalis* is a thin layer of fascia that lines the inner surface of the transversus abdominis muscle.

   Deep Inguinal Ring is an oval opening about 1.2 cm above the mid-inguinal point in the fascia transversalis.

   Internal spermatic fascia forms a tubular prolongation around the spermatic cord.

   Femoral sheath is the prolongation into the thigh over the femoral vessels.

   Iliopubic tract is the thickened inferior margin of the fascia transversalis in the inguinal region.

   Cremaster muscle fasciculi, embedded in the *cremasteric fascia*, are a series of U-shaped loops around the spermatic cord and testis. They are derived from internal oblique and transversus abdominis. It is fully developed in males but represented by few fibers in females.

7. Extraperitoneal tissue

8. Parietal peritoneum

Muscles of the Anterior Abdominal Wall

It constitutes five muscles that crisscross with each other and strengthen the abdominal wall, reducing the risk of hernias. Two vertical muscles, rectus and pyramidalis, are situated near the midline of the body, and three flat muscles, EO, IO, and TA, are located laterally and stacked on top of each other.

Development of Anterior Abdominal Muscles

The skeletal muscles are derived from the paraxial mesoderm. The abaxial muscle precursor cells differentiate into abdominal wall muscles in this region (the abaxial domain of mesoderm consists of a parietal layer of lateral plate mesoderm in combination with somite-derived cells that migrate in this region).

Rectus Sheath

It is an aponeurotic envelope for the rectus abdominis muscle on either side of the linea alba. It acts as a retinaculum for the rectus abdominis. It is derived from the aponeuroses of the tranversus abdominis, external and internal oblique. *Rectus Abdominis* with three or four tendinous horizontal intersections attached to the anterior wall of the rectus sheath. *Pyramidalis* is absent in nearly 20% of the population.

Inguinal Canal

It is an oblique passage (4 cm) in the lower part of the anterior abdominal wall, located just above the medial half of the ligament, which lodges the spermatic cord/round ligament of the uterus and ilioinguinal nerve. It extends from deep to the superficial inguinal ring.

Inguinal Triangle (Hesselbach's Triangle)

It is situated deep to the posterior wall of the inguinal canal. The peritoneum, extraperitoneal tissue, and fascia transversalis form the triangle floor.
  Boundaries

- *Medial*: Lower 5 cm of the lateral border of the rectus abdominis muscle.

- *Lateral*: Inferior epigastric artery.

- *Inferior*: Medial half of the inguinal ligament.

Urachus

The omphalomesenteric duct (connects the developing gut to the yolk sac), umbilical vessels, and urachus lie between the yolk sac and embryo. Urachus is a remnant of the cloaca (cranial continuation of urogenital sinus-fetal bladder precursor) and allantois (yolk sac derivative) at the umbilicus level. During gestation, urachus helps remove waste via the umbilical cord. Still, it gets obliterated within a few days of birth to remain as a fibrous cord (remnant as median umbilical ligament) in the preperitoneal space of Retzius between the descended bladder and the umbilicus. Umbilical arteries remain as medial umbilical ligaments on both sides of the urachus.

  Failure of involution results in a gamut of urachal variants/anomalies:

- *Patent Urachus/Fistula*: Tubular connection between the urinary bladder and umbilicus due to complete failure in obliteration.

- *Vesicourachal Diverticulum*: Persistent tissue at the bladder with no connection to the umbilicus.

- *Umbilical Polyp or Sinus*: Persistent tissue at the umbilicus with no connection to the bladder.

- *Urachal Cyst*: Patency along the midportion of the urachus with the tract closing at the umbilicus and bladder.

Hernias

External hernias refer to the prolapse of intestinal loops through an abdominal or pelvic wall defect. It can be groin, ventral, and diaphragmatic.

  Internal hernias refer to the protrusion of a viscera through peritoneal or mesenteric orifices/foramen (congenital due to anomalous peritoneal attachments/internal rotation or acquired after trauma, surgery, etc.) within the boundary of the peritoneal cavity.

  Major types of hernias are discussed in Table 8.6.

Table 8.6: **Major Types of Hernias**

External	Through abdominal wall opening
	Groin (Inguinal and femoral)
	Ventral (Anterior and lateral)
	Anterior (umbilical, paraumbilical, epigastric, and hypogastric)
	Lateral (Spigelian)
	Posterior (Lumbar)
Internal	Across mesenteric or peritoneal apertures
Diaphragmatic	Diaphragmatic weakness

Groin Hernias

- Inguinal

  a. *Direct*: Herniation through acquired weak defect in the posterior wall of the inguinal canal; passes medially to inferior epigastric vessels.

  b. *Indirect*: Most common: protrusion of peritoneal contents through patent internal inguinal ring lateral to inferior epigastric vessels and exits at external inguinal ring. The hernial extension is along the spermatic cord into the scrotum in males and the round ligament into the labia majora in females.

- *Femoral*: Less frequent; herniation through a congenital defect in transverse fascia attachment to the pubis; femoral canal lies medial to femoral vein below the inguinal ligament and lateral to pubic tubercle; with a high propensity to strangulation and incarceration.

Characteristic features of hernias are discussed in Table 8.7.

Table 8.7: **Characteristic Features of Hernias**

Umbilical	Midline; most common High risk of incarceration and strangulation
Paraumbilical	Through linea alba; a/w diastasis
Epigastric	Midline; above the level of umbilicus; on linea alba between the umbilicus and xiphoid process; contains properitoneal fat, vascular structure, and abdominal viscera rarely
Hypogastric	Midline; between umbilicus and pubic symphysis, prone to incarceration and strangulation
Spigelian	Posterior layer of transverse fascia along the linea semilunaris between rectus sheath and oblique muscles; arcuate line
Grynfeltt-Lesshaft	Due to a defect in the lumbar muscles/posterior fascia (between quadratus lumborum and oblique muscles) in the superior lumbar triangle
Petit's	Due to a defect between the quadratus lumborum and oblique muscles in the inferior lumbar triangle
Incisional	Usually midline and can be situated anywhere through any incision (vertical>transverse)or drain opening

Table 8.8 depicts the list of rare hernias.

Table 8.8: **List of Rare Hernias**

Ritcher's hernia	Antimesenteric bowel wall herniates
Maydl's hernia	Herniation of two small bowel loops (two afferent and efferent each) in the sac; prone to strangulation
Littre's (persistent omphalomesenteric duct) hernia	Meckel's diverticulum in inguinal hernia sac
Amyand's hernia	Appendix in inguinal hernia sac
Sciatic hernia	Small bowel/ureter herniates through the greater or lesser sciatic foramen
Obturator	Protrusion of peritoneal sac through the obturator foramen and extension between pectineal and obturator muscles
Perineal hernias	Elderly females' pelvic floor laxity

NORMAL VARIANTS

- *Prominent Lateral Arcuate Ligament*
  Mimics a retroperitoneal mass or peritoneal metastases in the hepatorenal pouch

- *Prominent Diaphragmatic Slips*
  Mimic peritoneal implants. But the prominent slips are curvilinear, contiguous with the diaphragm, and are separated from adjacent organs by fat. The expiratory phase helps delineate the variant.

- *Prominent Diaphragmatic Crus*
  Simulates retroperitoneal adenopathy

PATHOLOGY

Case 140 Mesenteric Panniculitis

A 40-year-old female with nonspecific abdominal pain (Figure 8.4).

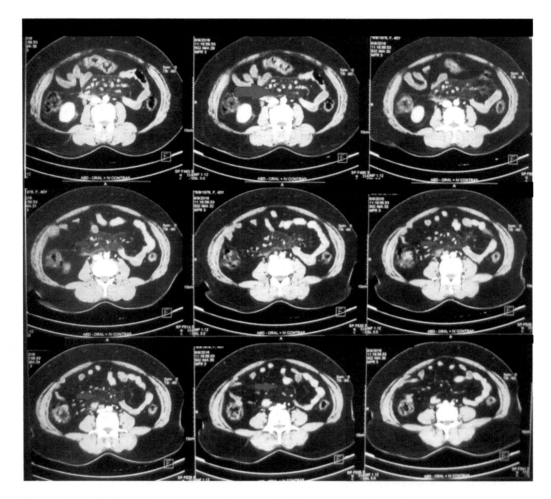

Figure 8.4 CECT abdomen depicts circumscribed hyperattenuating inflammatory mesenteric fat stranding (misty/hazy mesentery) with hypodense fatty halo (arrowhead) surrounding blood vessels and scattered nodules along with peripheral soft tissue attenuation rim surrounding the inflammatory mesenteric mass (pseudo capsule).

Discussion

Mesenteric panniculitis is characterized by nonspecific inflammation of the subcutaneous adipose tissue within small bowel mesentery, predominantly in the jejunal mesentery. It is frequent in males with a history of prior trauma, surgery, cancer, or any autoimmune disease.

Three stages

- Mesenteric lipodystrophy (fat degeneration)

- Mesenteric panniculitis (inflammation)

- Sclerosing/retractile mesenteritis (SM—ill-defined infiltration with calcification, fibrosis, and retraction of surrounding structures)

CECT reveals

- Vessels and scattered soft tissue density nodules in the hyperattenuating tumor-like mesenteric enlargement with local mass effect displacing the bowel loops regionally
- Hyperdense fibrotic rim of pseudocapsule encasing the lesion
- Hypodense halo of fat around the vessels (fat halo sign)

Sonography shows well-defined heterogeneously hyperechoic mass. MRI reveals T1 hypo/intermediate intensity and T2 hyperintense mass in the inflammatory form of mesenteric panniculitis. Sclerosing form is hypointense on both T1- and T2WI. Pseudocapsule is hypointense, and fibrous tissue shows delayed contrast enhancement and no restriction on DWI.

Differential Diagnosis

1. Mesenteric edema (in patients with ascites and systemic diseases such as cirrhosis, renal failure, pancreatitis, appendicitis, etc.)
2. Mesenteric hemorrhage (iatrogenic/traumatic; hyperintense on T1WI)
3. Lymphoma (ill-defined mesenteric fat infiltration with enlarged coalescent LAP)
4. Well-differentiated liposarcoma
5. Peritoneal TB—multiple mesenteric nodularity, peritoneal thickening, necrotic LAP, and ascites)
6. Carcinoid tumor (a/w hypervascular bowel tumor with hepatic metastasis), desmoid, and peritoneal carcinomatosis mimic sclerosing/retractile mesenteritis

Management

Steroids and follow-up CT for interval changes.

Case 141 Richter Hernia

A 70-year-old female presented with abdominal pain and vomiting (Figure 8.5).

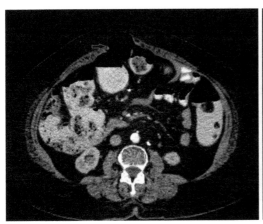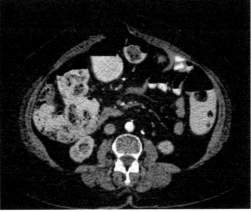

Figure 8.5   CECT abdomen depicts focal protrusion of the antimesenteric wall of a bowel loop into a small defect in the abdominal wall.

Discussion

Richter hernia, named after German surgeon August Gottlieb Richter, is a herniation of the anti-mesenteric part of the circumference of the bowel wall through the minor fascial defect. It is commonly noted in elderly females and may present abdominal distention, nausea, and vomiting. Common locations include femoral canal > inguinal canal > abdominal wall incisional hernia (due to unclosed port sites following laparoscopic or robotic-assisted surgeries). It may present as chronic incarceration or enterocutaneous fistula if not appropriately managed.

Differentials

- Lipomas

- Abscesses

- Bowel obstruction due to adhesions, etc.

Management

Surgery

Case 142 Gossypiboma

A 42-year-old female with abdominal pain, fever, and a history of surgery (Figure 8.6).

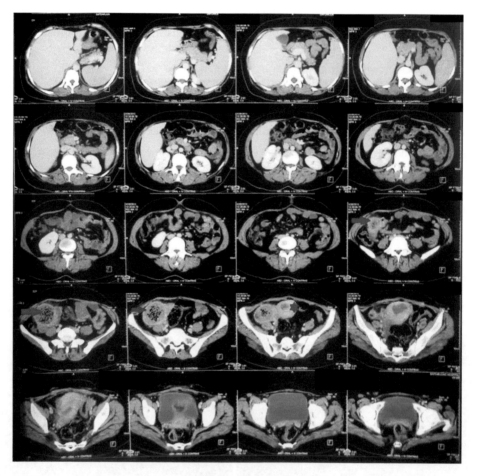

Figure 8.6 CECT abdomen reveals multiple air foci within an encapsulated hypodense mass with wall enhancement in the right lower abdomen adjacent to bowel loops and an enlarged uterus with endometrial collection (star).

Discussion

Gossypiboma (textiloma) refers to retained surgical sponge, often a/w prolonged or emergency surgery, unexpected hemorrhage, or inadequate number/inexperienced/change of staff during the surgery. This foreign body results in

- *Acute Reaction*: Exudative inflammatory reaction with abscess/fistula formation. Over the years, the fistulous tract may form externally via the abdominal wall or internally to the intestine (migration causing intestinal obstruction), bladder, or vagina and may result in the extrusion of the foreign body.

- *Delayed Reaction*: Fibrinous aseptic inflammatory reaction with adhesions, encapsulation/granuloma formation.

Patients may present with pain, vomiting, fever, and abdominal distension. Sonography reveals thick-walled complex cystic lesions with curvy hyperechoic areas, gas bubbles, and posterior dirty shadowing. CECT may have varied presentations—a heterogeneous collection with rim enhancement, spongiform pattern with gas bubbles, or cystic lesion with thick calcified rind and reticulate pattern. On angiography, a gossypiboma may appear as a hypervascular tumor.

Differentials

- Hemostatic agents (bioabsorbable materials) control intraoperative bleeding that is kept intentionally during surgery (tightly packed air foci compared to scattered air foci and thick enhancing capsule in gossypiboma).

- Abscess, tumors, etc.

Management

Surgery

Case 143 Intraperitoneal Hydatid

A 29-year-old patient with abdominal discomfort (Figure 8.7).

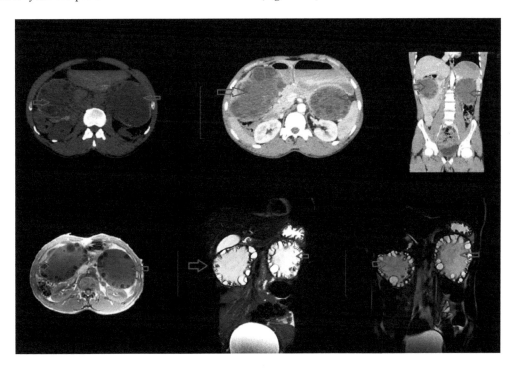

Figure 8.7 CT (upper row) depicts well-defined, thin-walled cysts with peripherally located daughter cysts in the peritoneal cavity. MRI (lower row) reveals hydatid cysts as low SI on T1WI and high SI on T2WI with a hypointense rim of pericyst on both T1WI and T2WI. Daughter cysts appear relatively more hypointense on T1WI and hyperintense on T2WI.

Discussion

Peritoneal seeding is mainly caused by hepatic hydatid disease secondary to traumatic or surgical rupture of the hepatic or splenic echinococcal cyst or asymptomatic micro ruptures into the peritoneal cavity. Sporadic cases of primary peritoneal hydatidosis have been reported rarely.

Multiple cysts of varying sizes can be found anywhere in the peritoneal cavity. Most people are asymptomatic for several years. Enlarging abdominal cysts may cause nonspecific symptoms such as abdominal discomfort, anorexia, vomiting, and dyspepsia. A ruptured cyst in the peritoneum may cause acute abdominal pain or acute allergic symptoms if the antigenic fluid has been released into the peritoneal cavity and absorbed into the circulation.

Hydatid cysts can be seen clearly on ultrasound, CT, and MRI. Multiple cysts can form anywhere in the peritoneal cavity. Peritoneal echinococcus can sometimes encompass the entire peritoneal cavity, simulating a multiloculated mass known as encysted peritoneal hydatidosis.

The appearance of hydatid cysts on imaging is similar to that of hepatic disease, as discussed in Chapter 1.

Case 144 Pneumoperitoneum

A 32-year-old patient with abdominal discomfort (Figure 8.8).

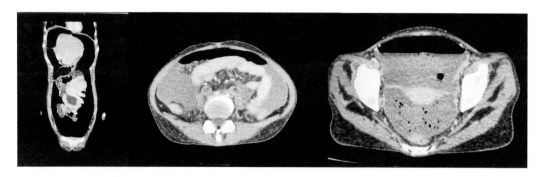

Figure 8.8 CECT abdomen depicts multiple air foci along the anterior and anterolateral abdominal wall, perihepatic space, right perirenal, lienorenal space, and pelvic cavity s/o pneumoperitoneum. Gross ascites noted.

Discussion

Pneumoperitoneum is termed as the presence of free intraperitoneal air, the most common causes being hollow viscus perforation, trauma, postoperatively or iatrogenic (peritoneal dialysis, endoscopy, post-intubation or mechanical ventilation).

Upright Chest X-rays and decubitus abdominal X-rays can detect free air. Experienced sonographers can identify free intraperitoneal air as enhanced peritoneal stripe echogenicity that changes position with a change in the patient's position apart from reverberation echoes. Trapped air bubbles in the fluid collection appear as echogenic foci. CT scan suggests the importance of switching to lung and bone windows and is crucial in delineating the cause and extent of pneumoperitoneum.

Differentials

- Pseudopneumoperitoneum due to Chiladiti syndrome, gas within skin folds, subdiaphragmatic and properitoneal fat.

- *Pneumoretroperitoneum*: Free air surrounds kidneys, great vessels, duodenum, and pancreas apart from.

- *Tension Pneumoperitoneum*: Free air is under pressure due to the ball-valve effect.

- Abdominal compartment syndrome.

Management

- Spontaneous pneumoperitoneum that does not involve hollow viscous perforation is managed conservatively.

- Perforation peritonitis is managed by immediate exploratory laparotomy.

Case 145 Ventral Hernia

A 48-year-old patient with hernia (Figure 8.9).

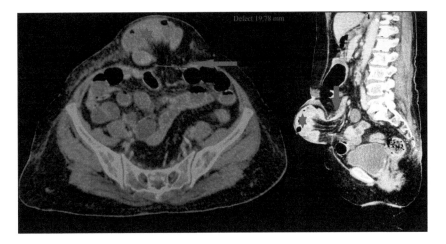

Figure 8.9 CECT abdomen depicts an anterior abdominal wall defect (solid arrow) in the hypogastric region through which omental fat and bowel loops (star) herniate.

Discussion

Hernias occur due to protrusion of contents through congenital or acquired weakness secondary to surgery, trauma, or defects in the musculoskeletal system. Risk factors include female gender, mutiparity, aging, obesity, ascites, and large intraabdominal masses. It could be primary and incisional. It can be reducible (disappears spontaneously/with external pressure), irreducible (incarcerated), obstructed (with small bowel obstruction), and strangulated (compromised vascular supply) may occur. CT precisely evaluates the site, size, extent, and contents of the hernia, along with complications, if any.

Differential

Rectus diastasis—protrusion of fat/bowel through the gap (> 2 cm) between right and left recti muscles, without any fascial defect.

Management

Surgery, depending on the presentation.

Case 146 Femoral Hernia

A 48-year-old female with lower abdominal discomfort and bulge (Figure 8.10).

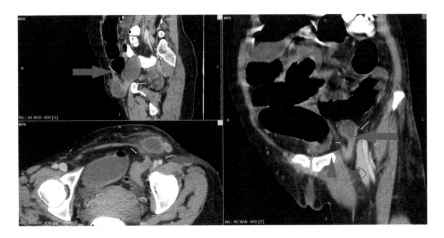

Figure 8.10 CECT abdomen depicts femoral hernia lateral to pubic tubercle (arrowhead) and medial to the common femoral vein (open arrow).

Discussion

Femoral hernia is a protrusion of a peritoneal sac through the femoral ring into the femoral canal, posteroinferior to the inguinal ligament, lateral to pubic tubercle, medial to common femoral vein, inferior to inferior epigastric vessels. This narrow-necked hernia may cause engorgement of distal collateral veins due to compression of femoral veins. Right-sided hernias are more common. Femoral hernias are prone to incarceration.

Differentials

- Inguinal hernias, in comparison, lie medial to the pubic tubercle and are common in males.

- Obturator hernias through obturator canal.

Management

Surgery

Case 147 Poliomyelitis with Kyphoscoliosis and Hydronephrosis

A 20-year-old female with poliomyelitis (Figure 8.11).

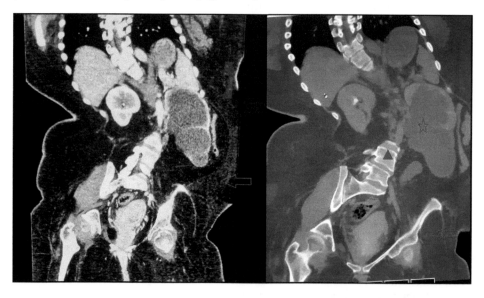

Figure 8.11 CT abdomen depicts severely reduced bulk (arrow) of left-sided muscles around the hip, proximal thigh, and anterior abdominal wall muscles in a patient with poliomyelitis. Severe kyphoscoliotic deformity (arrowhead) with curvature toward the left side. Enlarged left kidney with abrupt termination of distal ureter and mild periureteric fat stranding resulting in severe upstream hydroureteronephrosis (star) and thinning of renal parenchyma in the non-excretory left kidney (no excretion even on delayed scans).

Discussion

Poliomyelitis, a vaccine-preventable viral disease with fecal-oral transmission, results in morbid paralytic disability due to the destruction of motor neurons. Patients present with progressive muscle weakness, myalgias, respiratory distress, joint pain, atrophy, dysphagia, and generalized fatigue. Imaging depicts fat/muscle/bony atrophy along with deformities of bones and joints such as contractures, scoliosis, etc.

Management

- General supportive measures. Surgical management, orthoses, and exercise programs for physical rehabilitation.

- Ureteric stricture is noted as a smooth tapering of the transition zone requiring ureteroscopy for management.

Case 148 Pseudomyxoma Peritonei Due to Mucinous Neoplasm of the Appendix
A 60-year-old female with abdominal distension and weight loss (Figure 8.12).

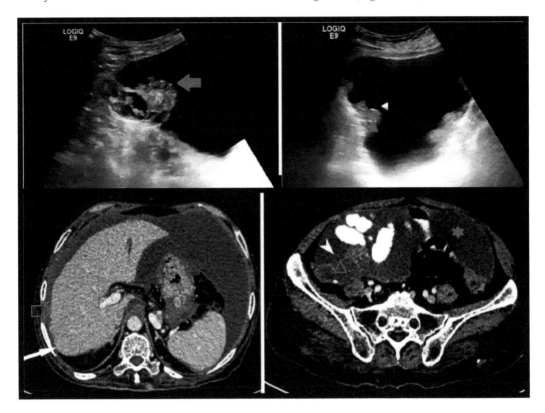

Figure 8.12 Sonography reveals a heterogenous lesion (solid arrow) with calcific foci in the RIF region and ascites (star) with peritoneal deposits (arrowhead). CECT abdomen showing liver scalloping (open arrow) and spleen parenchyma with ascites. Mixed density lesion in RIF region arising from the ileocecal region (arrowhead).

Discussion

Pseudomyxoma peritonei is a rare entity developed due to mucinous ascites caused by rupture of the mucinous neoplasm, the mucinous adenocarcinoma of the appendix being the most common cause, followed by neoplasms of the ovary. It is relatively more common in females. Imaging shows ascites with non-mobile echogenic particles/simple or loculated hypodense fluid. Omental thickening, and enhancing peritoneal deposits were also noted.

Differentials

- Pseudomyxoma peritonei due to ovarian neoplasm (raised CA-125 levels)
- Peritoneal carcinomatosis
- Peritonitis

Management

Surgical debulking +/– chemotherapy (systemic/intraperitoneal)

Case 149 Retroperitoneal Abscess Secondary to Ruptured Appendix
A 19-year-old male with right-sided pain and fever (Figure 8.13).

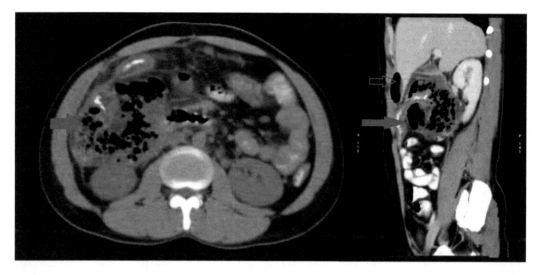

Figure 8.13 CECT abdomen depicts a large, well-defined, peripherally enhancing multiloculated collection showing air foci within, noted in the right pararenal space with inflamed and edematous adjacent caecum, ascending colon up to hepatic flexure. Retrocaecal appendix with indistinct wall suggests rupture. A lentiform peripherally enhancing collection showing air-fluid level along the anterior surface of the liver (peri-hepatic abscess).

Discussion

Atypical signs and symptoms, a delayed diagnosis, a higher risk of perforation, and severe complications such as empyema, portomesenteric thrombosis, and abscesses in the retroperitoneum, liver, scrotum, thigh, and lumbar region are a/w ruptured retrocaecal appendicitis.

Retroperitoneal abscess is an uncommon and dangerous complication of retrocecal appendicitis. However, it can also develop as a complication of other diseases like diverticulitis, pancreatitis, pyelonephritis, perforation of colonic carcinoma, etc. The presence of an inflamed appendix with an indistinct wall suggests rupture. A plain abdominal X-ray may show obliteration of psoas shadow or gas bubbles overlying the right abdominal wall. CT better delineates the extent of focal collection/abscess with air foci and helps plan treatment.

Management

Urgent laparotomy and intravenous antibiotics

Case 150 Retroperitoneal Sarcoma

A 54-year-old patient with backache and abdominal discomfort (Figure 8.14).

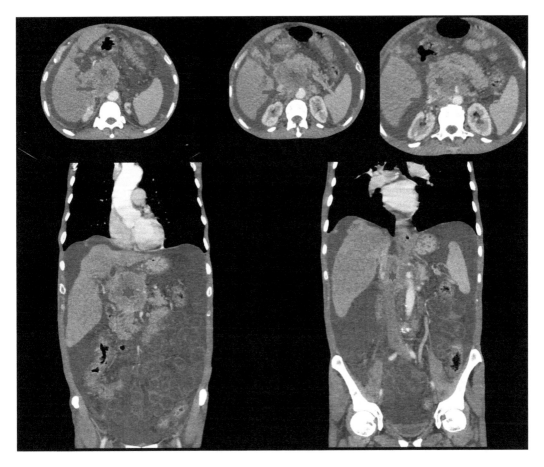

Figure 8.14 CECT abdomen reveals an ill-defined heterogeneously enhancing hypoattenuat-ing soft tissue density lesion in the retroperitoneal region in the vascular compartment infiltrat-ing distal CBD (upstream proximal dilatation), caudate lobe of liver, extrahepatic portal vein, and infra-hepatic IVC, celiac trunk, superior mesenteric vessels, pancreatic head, and liver with metas-tasis (open arrow), collaterals, and gross ascites—retroperitoneal sarcoma with metastasis.

Discussion

Retroperitoneal sarcomas are aggressive, multifocal, malignant mesenchymal tumors, the com-mon types being liposarcomas, leiomyosarcomas, and undifferentiated soft tissue sarcomas, with a poor prognosis due to high rates of recurrence and distant spread.

The patient may be asymptomatic or the presentation depends on its size, location, and growth pattern (compression/encasement of adjacent structures).

CECT reveals heterogeneous lesions (in the retroperitoneal cavity) with necrotic areas that appear heterogeneously hypointense on T1WI and hyperintense on T2WI. CT Chest should be done to look for lung metastasis. Image-guided percutaneous needle biopsy helps determine the need and extent of surgery.

Differentials

1. *Lymphoma*: a/w fever, night sweats, and weight loss. Obstruction of retroperitoneal lymphatics resulting in leakage of chyle (chylous ascites).

2. Malignant primary (testicular) tumor metastasizing to retroperitoneum.

3. Liposarcomas (macroscopic fat content with negative HU on CT, high signal on T1WI, and signal loss on fat-suppressed sequences).

4. Leiomyosarcoma usually arises from vessels, mainly IVC.

Management

Surgery

Case 151 Urachal Adenocarcinoma

A 55-year-old male with foul-smelling discharge from anterior abdominal wall growth and weight loss (Figure 8.15).

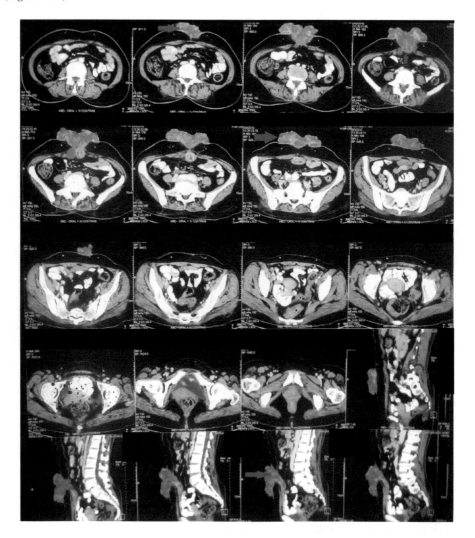

Figure 8.15 CECT abdomen depicts an exophytic lesion arising from the anterior wall and dome of the urinary bladder, infiltrating the anterior abdominal wall musculature with loss of fat planes and extending up to the skin.

Discussion

Urachal adenocarcinoma, a rare entity frequently found in elderly males, usually midline, infra umbilical location, presents as hematuria, dysuria, abdominal pain, etc. Bladder adenocarcinoma is usually a/w persistent urachus, urinary diversions, and bladder exstrophy. It occurs due to malignant transformation of columnar epithelium. The lesion is initially silent and presents at an advanced stage after invasion to adjacent structures.

Imaging shows heterogeneous solid-cystic growth involving the anterior abdominal wall and urinary bladder dome. Cystic components represent mucin. Calcific foci may be seen. The lesion is hyperintense on T2WI due to mucinous or necrotic components. The lesion is isointense on T1WI and shows contrast enhancement. The lesion may metastasize to lymph nodes, lungs, etc.

Differentials

- Infected urachal remnant
- Benign urachal tumors
- Primary bladder adenocarcinoma (Extravesical component is more in urachal adenocarcinoma)

Management

- Surgical excision (cystectomy with urachal mass resection)
- Chemo/radiotherapy

PEDIATRIC

Case 152 Congenital Diaphragmatic Hernia

An infant with respiratory distress (Figure 8.16).

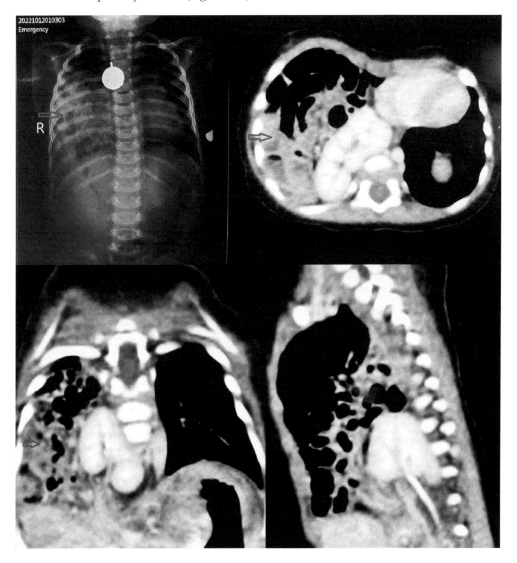

Figure 8.16   CXR shows indistinct right hemidiaphragm multiple bowel loops herniated in the right hemithorax, causing contralateral mediastinal shift. CT depicts a large defect in the postero-lateral aspect of the right hemidiaphragm with the herniation of small and large bowel loops and right kidney in the right thoracic cavity with contralateral mediastinal shift.

Discussion

By the ninth week of pregnancy, diaphragmatic development is typically completed. Congenital diaphragmatic hernias (CDHs) develop when one of the pleuroperitoneal canals fails to fuse at around 8 weeks—a developmental defect in the diaphragm results in the herniation of abdominal contents into the thoracic cavity. Most commonly, the defects are left posterolateral (Bochdalek's hernia-70%–80%), and sometimes the right anteromedial region (Morgagni's hernia 15%–20%) is involved. Central hernias are rare. Left-sided CDH frequently presents with herniation of the stomach and intestines with peristalsis and contralateral mediastinal shift to the right. A portion of the liver can be seen in the chest with right-sided CDH. Additional landmarks could include the position of the gall bladder or the doppler examinations of the umbilical vein and hepatic vasculature. Antenatal sonography and fetal MRI are beneficial in assessing the hernia and associated conditions. Observed/expected lung-to-head ratio (o/e LHR) to assess lung size by sonography predicts survival in patients with CDH. Isolated CDH has a better prognosis than if associated with pulmonary hypoplasia and various renal, cardiac, gastrointestinal, and nervous system anomalies. The infant may present with respiratory distress, cyanosis, barrel-shaped chest, scaphoid abdomen, absent breath sounds, shifted cardiac sounds, and bowel sounds in the chest.

Antenatal sonography of CDH

- Abdominal organs such as the stomach (left-sided defects) usually behind the left heart and liver (right-sided defects) in the thorax

- Bowel peristalsis in the thorax

- Small abdominal circumference

- Polyhydramnios

- Doppler study corroborates the course of abnormally positioned elongated vessels

Differential Diagnosis

- Intrathoracic lesions such as congenital cystic adenomatoid malformation, loculated pneumothorax, and bronchopulmonary sequestration

- Diaphragmatic eventration

Management

- Fetal endoscopic tracheal occlusion occludes the trachea with a balloon from about 26 weeks to 34 weeks of gestation to increase fetal lung fluid/volume to promote lung growth.

- Intubation and corrective surgery when the neonate is physiologically stable, usually within a week of delivery.

Case 153 Urachal Cyst

A 15-year-old girl for abdominal pain (Figure 8.17).

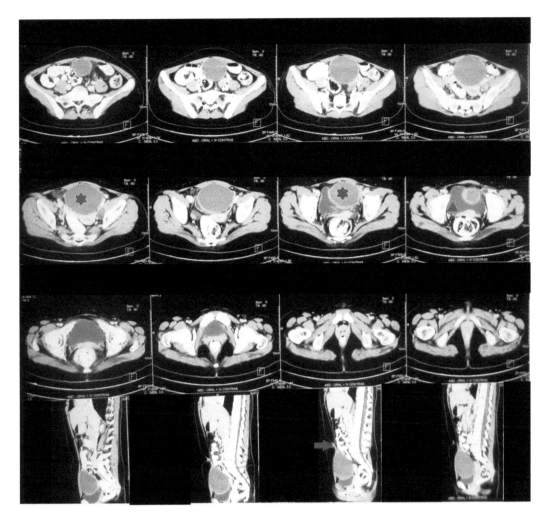

Figure 8.17   CECT abdomen depicts a cystic lesion (star) anterior and contiguous with the bladder (arrowhead) dome extending toward the umbilicus (arrow) along the course of the urachal remnant.

Discussion

Urachal cyst is an extraperitoneal fluid density lesion noted in the anterior abdominal wall (umbilical region). It is usually asymptomatic unless infected and presents with abdominal pain, fever, or ruptures, resulting in peritonitis. Malignancy may develop in some cases. Closure of both the umbilical and bladder ends of urachus results in the formation of urachal cysts.

Differentials

- Umbilical sebaceous cyst/hernia
- Vitelline cyst
- Mesenteric cyst

Management

Surgical excision

Case 154 Bladder Exstrophy

Male child with birth defect (Figure 8.18).

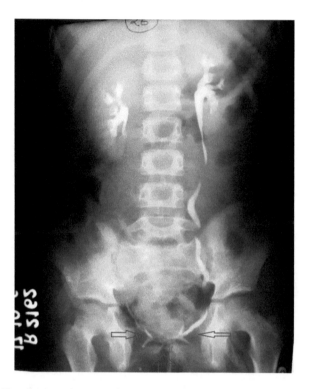

Figure 8.18 IVP film depicts absent pubic symphysis, widely separated pubic bones, non-visualized urinary bladder, laterally, and upward angulated bilateral ureters at UVJ. Normal bilateral kidneys.

Discussion

Bladder exstrophy (ectopia vesicae), a congenital anomaly, refers to deficient midline closure of the infraumbilical region of the anterior abdominal wall with absent rectus muscles (deficient transverse, internal oblique, and external oblique muscles) resulting in urinary bladder eversion outside the pelvic cavity. The bladder appears solid (not cystic as in the pelvic cavity normally) as it is not filled by the bilateral ureters, which void directly into the amniotic cavity.

Antenatal sonography shows a non-visualized bladder even after repeat scans, normal amniotic fluid volume, normal kidneys and ureters, abdominal wall mass below a low umbilical cord insertion, anomalous genitalia, and widely separated pubic bones. Genital abnormalities include cryptorchidism, inguinal hernia, or short stubby penis curved upwards (epispadias) in males and short urethra buried in everted bladder, bifid clitoris, widely separated labia, short stenotic vagina, and uterine prolapse in females. IVP and MRI further corroborate the diagnosis and help in surgical planning.

Differentials on Antenatal Sonography

- Temporary absent bladder on antenatal sonography: Repeat the scan in 30 minutes.
- Renal malformations (bilateral renal agenesis, PCKD, and MCDK): Kidneys are abnormal, and amniotic fluid is low.
- *Placental Insufficiency*: Fetal growth restriction with oligohydramnios.

Management

Surgery for genitalia and bladder reconstruction or urinary diversion

SUGGESTED READINGS

Eren, S., & Çiriş, F. Diaphragmatic hernia: Diagnostic approaches with review of the literature. *Eur J Radiol.* 2005;54(3):448–459. doi: 10.1016/j.ejrad.2004.09.008.

Healy, J., & Reznek, R. The peritoneum, mesenteries and omenta: Normal anatomy and pathological processes. *Eur Radiol.* 1998;8:886–900. doi: 10.1007/s003300050485.

Tirkes, T., Sandrasegaran, K., Patel, A. A., Hollar, M. A., Tejada, J. G., Tann, M., Akisik, F. M., & Lappas, J. C. Peritoneal and etroperitoneal anatomy and its relevance for cross-sectional imaging. *Radiographics* 2012;32:2, 437–451.

Yu, J.-S., Kim, K. W., Lee, H.-J., Lee, Y.-J., Yoon, C.-S., & Kim, M.-J. Urachal remnant diseases: Spectrum of CT and US findings. *Radiographics* 2001;21:2, 451–461.

9 Abdominal Tuberculosis and Role of AI in Abdominopelvic Radiology

SPECTRUM OF TUBERCULOSIS

Despite significant improvements in detection and treatment, tuberculosis (TB) remains among the most common causes of morbidity and mortality in developing nations. Significant morbidity can be prevented by receiving early diagnosis and treatment. A negative result from a skin test for tuberculin does not mean that TB is absent.

Abdominopelvic TB is a challenging condition to diagnose as the clinical and radiologic characteristics of tuberculosis also closely mimic those of numerous other illnesses. Intestinal TB frequently occurs as a sequela of latent TB reactivation or ingestion of tuberculous bacteria via unpasteurized milk, undercooked meat, or infected lung secretions apart from hematogeneous or lymphatic spread. Malnutrition, vitamin D deficiency, along with smokers, alcoholics, intravenous drug users, and patients on steroids and co-existing diseases (such as HIV, diabetes, renal failure, immunosuppression, liver failure, lung diseases, lymphomas, and malignancy) are at risk for increased propensity for tuberculosis and morbidity.

Imaging techniques are valuable for early detection, accurate diagnosis, and disease monitoring. Given this, radiologists and doctors must be familiar with tuberculosis's common signs and imaging patterns to diagnose it correctly. It should be considered a differential diagnosis for any patient with a fever of unknown origin, weight loss, or chronic abdominal discomfort. All suspicious patients should have a sputum analysis and a chest X-ray to look for other abnormalities. Ultrasound is essential for making diagnoses and providing guidance during surgical procedures. Early intervention can improve patient outcomes, assess treatment response, and prevent disease progression. Regular follow-up imaging can help ensure effective treatment and promptly detect any disease recurrence.

In summary, imaging is pivotal in managing abdominopelvic tuberculosis by aiding in early diagnosis, assessing disease extent, guiding interventions, and monitoring treatment response. It allows healthcare professionals to make informed decisions and provide timely and appropriate care to patients with this challenging form of tuberculosis.

Table 9.1 depicts imaging characteristics and differential diagnosis of tuberculosis affecting various body parts.

Table 9.1: Imaging Characteristics and Differential Diagnosis of Tuberculosis Affecting Various Body Parts

Organ	Sonography	CT/MRI	Differential Diagnoses
Peritoneal	Wet Peritonitis: Free or septated ascites. Fibrous peritonitis: Large omentum and mesenteric masses with fixed intestinal loops. Dry peritonitis Irregular mesenteric wall thickening, matted lymph nodes with caseous necrosis	Ascites Smooth & regular peritoneal thickening with marked enhancement on CECT. Hyperdense mesenteric root fat planes Enlarged necrotic/calcified lymph nodes	• Peritoneal carcinomatosis (irregular, multinodular thickening) • Peritoneal pseudomyxoma • Amyloidosis • Peritoneal mesothelioma • Lymphoma
Intestinal The ileocaecal (IC) region is the most frequently affected area due to stasis and lack of lymphatic tissue.	1. Concentric mural thickening of the caecum and the ileum with narrowing (strictures) of small bowel loops with proximal dilatation 2. Absence of peristalsis 3. Raised mesenteric echogenicity and thickness.	1. Abdominal CT is the best for assessing intra- and extraluminal involvement. 2. Asymmetrical thickening of the ileocecal region and the medial wall of the colon, with or without proximal intestinal dilatation	Crohn's disease (increased mesenteric vascularity, skip lesions, fistulas more common) Cecal malignancy Intestinal lymphoma Amebiasis CMLNS These entities do not present with ascites.

(Continued)

Table 9.1: (*Continued*) Imaging Characteristics and Differential Diagnosis of Tuberculosis Affecting Various Body Parts

Organ	Sonography	CT/MRI	Differential Diagnoses
	4. An IC region may retract into the subhepatic area, giving a pseudokidney sign 5. Sonography also helps guide paracentesis and lymph node aspiration for confirmatory diagnosis.	3. Non-specific findings include ascites, surrounding fat-stranding, necrotic lymphadenopathies, and omental thickening.	
Lymphnodes (mesenteric, periportal, peri-pancreatic, aortocaval, and retroperitoneal)	LNs appear matted, conglomerated, and hypoechoic with a more hypoechoic core due to caseation may calcify in late stages	1. Hypodense with homogenous enhancement (initially) or peripheral enhancement (due to caseation as the disease progresses) on CECT. 2. LNs may appear hypointense on T2 due to the presence of free radicals and central caseation necrosis and surrounding soft tissue edema	• Pyogenic infection • Lymphoma • Metastasis • Mesenteric lymphadenitis • CMLNS
Liver Spleen	Hepatosplenomegaly Diffuse increase in echogenicity and multiple hypoechoic or echogenic nodules. Linear high-frequency transducer is used for focal, hypoattenuating splenic microabscesses. Granulomas and periportal hypoechoic masses coexist with dispersed foci of calcifications. Calcifications may be identified in chronic forms	Multiple peripherally enhancing, hypodense lesions of varying sizes. Lymphadenopathy, ascites, and calcifications in later stages. Lesions are hypointense on T1WI, iso/hyperintense on T2WI with peripheral enhancement, and restricted diffusion on DWI.	*Miliary form* Metastasis Lymphoma Sarcoidosis Fungal infection *Macronodular form* Pyogenic abscess Malignancy
Adrenal Rare, bilateral but asymmetrical. Clinically resembles Addison's disease because of progressive destruction of both glands		Acute and subacute stages 1. Diffuse and homogenously enlarged gland or a hypodense core with peripheral enhancement. 2. A solid mass with preserved glandular contours suggests granulomatous disease rather than neoplasia Chronic stages Reduced gland size with calcifications	Metastasis Lymphoma Primary neoplasia Hemorrhage
Pancreas	Focal Ill-defined hypoechoic mass Diffuse Gland size enlargement with or without stenosis of the main pancreatic duct	Low-attenuation, peripherally-enhancing mass. Calcifications in chronic stages.	Pyogenic abscess Hypodense lesions of pancreas (Table 1.25)

(*Continued*)

201

Table 9.1: (*Continued*) Imaging Characteristics and Differential Diagnosis of Tuberculosis Affecting Various Body Parts

Organ	Sonography	CT/MRI	Differential Diagnoses
Urinary Tract Patient presents with hematuria, chronic dysuria, and frequent urination. The hallmark of TB is the involvement of multiple sites and different stages of diseases like granulomas, cavitation, fibrosis, and calcification seen in the same patient.	1. Varied grades of hydronephrosis 2. Urothelial thickening of the renal pelvis, 3. Pyonephrosis (hydronephrosis with echogenic and moving debris) 4. Occasionally, renal abscesses may rupture and extend into the perinephric space. Healing occurs through fibrosis and calcification. This progression of fibrosis results in the scarred cortex, a pulled-up ureter with vesicoureteral reflux, and, eventually, autonephrectomy.	CECT is sometimes impossible due to abnormal kidney function. However, urine smear and culture with cystoscopic biopsy are diagnostic. 1. Moth-eaten calyces Parenchymal mass, amputated infundibula, autonephrectomy, thickening of urinary tract walls, parenchymal and cavity calcifications, cavities in the renal parenchyma, hydrocalcinosis, hydronephrosis, and hydroureter secondary to segmental stenosis. The ureter may appear dilated due to the stenotic areas or vesicoureteral reflux, secondary to bacilluria. Multiple strictures resulting in uneven caliectasis. Healed/chronic: Renal atrophy, progressive hydronephrosis, and dystrophic calcifications ("putty kidney"). Multiple extensive calcifications in the ureteral tract (pipeline ureter). Imaging findings include thickening, mural irregularity and calcifications, reduced bladder capacity (thimble bladder) and ulcers.	*Kidneys* Pyogenic infection Papillary necrosis Malignancy *Ureter* Ureteric strictures due to other benign and malignant etiologies *Bladder* Chemo/radiotherapy-induced cystitis Malignancy
Genital tract Fallopian tubes (presents with infertility) and endometrium	Echogenic particles in the pelvic space ascites Thickened irregular walls of tubo-ovarian abscess Hydrosalpinx Tubal block. Irregularly thickened and heterogeneous endometrium with/ without free air and fluid in cul de sac. Saline infusion sonohysterography SIS (irregular endometrial contour with a scarred uterine cavity; to check tubal patency).		*Tubo-ovarian* Pyogenic abscesses Malignancy *Endometrium* Endometritis (bacterial/fungal infection or instrumentation) Uterine adhesions Endometrial carcinoma
Male genital tract (epididymis is the most common site due to rich blood supply)	Transrectal ultrasound scan (TRUS) Multiple focal hypoechoic areas, calcifications, and abscesses in the prostate. Anourethral fistula with air shadowing.	CT showed hypodense lesions associated with necrotic areas, hyperenhancement, and peripheral calcifications.	Pyogenic lesions Malignancy

(Continued)

Table 9.1: (*Continued*) Imaging Characteristics and Differential Diagnosis of Tuberculosis Affecting Various Body Parts

Organ	Sonography	CT/MRI	Differential Diagnoses
	Multiple epididymal cysts or a diffusely enlarged heterogeneous hypoechoic region with hyperemia and dilated seminal vesicles with or without calcifications Tuberculous orchitis show enlarged testis with small hypoechoic nodules, blurred testis-epididymis interface, diffuse hypoechoic enlargement, sinus tract formation and scrotal abscesses.	MRI showed increased gland volume with a "watermelon" sign on T2, where the gland appears hypointense with high-signal striations, although this appearance is nonspecific.	
Soft Tissue (paravertebral area or iliopsoas muscle)-Pott's disease	Sonography-guided drainage for treating the infection apart from anti-tubercular therapy.	Calcifications within the abscess are highly suggestive of TB.	Pyogenic/fungal abscesses Soft tissue tumors

Case 155 Peritoneal Tuberculosis

A 48-year-old male patient presented with RLQ pain, vomiting, loss of appetite, and weight loss for the last 2 months. Investigations revealed raised ESR (Figure 9.1).

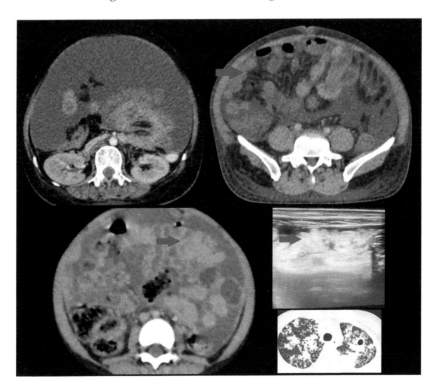

Figure 9.1   CECT and sonography abdomen depict ascites (star), peritoneal and omental thickening with smudged/cake appearance (arrow) in a patient with pulmonary tuberculosis (arrowhead).

Discussion

Peritoneal tuberculosis, involving the peritoneum, mesentery, and omentum, is the most frequent presentation of abdominal TB with dissemination to adjacent lymph nodes and organs. Patients may present with abdominal pain, asthenia, low-grade fever, night sweats, vomiting, alternating diarrhea and constipation, anorexia, weight loss, and right iliac fossa mass, depending on the region involved. Abdomino-pelvic infection spreads through the hematogenous route apart from lymphatic spread and via ingestion of mycobacterium. All HIV-positive individuals presenting with fever, unexplained weight loss, weakness, diarrhea, or abdominal pain should be evaluated for disseminated abdominal TB, as discussed in Table 9.1.

Any of the following criteria can confirm the diagnosis:

1. Presence of acid-fast bacilli in tissue or fluid.

2. Presence of caseation necrosis in the tissue specimen.

3. Characteristic granulomas or chronic inflammatory infiltrate and epitheloid cells on histology.

4. Ascitic fluid analysis—lymphocytic; low serum ascites albumin gradient; high adenosine deaminase ascites.

5. WHO currently recommends only the Xpert® MTB/RIF assay for diagnosing TB. It can provide results within 2 hours. Nevertheless, negative results cannot rule out the disease.

Imaging findings are not pathognomonic but may highly suggest the disease in conjunction with clinical and laboratory findings.

Management

Antitubercular therapy

Case 156 Tubercular Lymphadenitis

A 35-year-old patient with pulmonary tuberculosis (Figure 9.2).

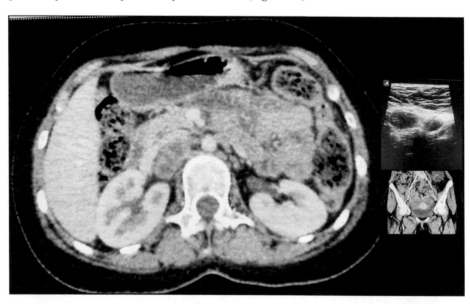

Figure 9.2 Sonography and CECT abdomen depict necrotic lymph nodes in the retroperitoneum and the pelvic cavity.

Discussion

Sonography shows enlarged hypoechoic lymph nodes with a matted/conglomerated pattern. Early nodes show homogeneous enhancement. With caseation necrosis, lymph nodes become heterogeneous and show peripheral rim enhancement. Healed tuberculosis in the later stages shows calcifications.

Management

Antitubercular therapy

Case 157 Tubercular Liver Abscess

A 25-year-old male k/c/o tuberculosis (Figure 9.3).

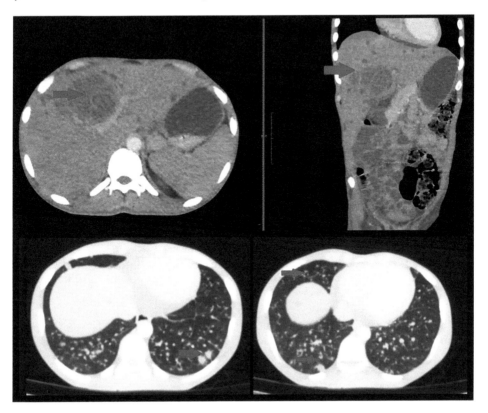

Figure 9.3 CECT abdomen depicts hepatomegaly with a large ill-defined multiloculated peripherally enhancing hypodense collection with indistinct margins showing multiple irregular enhancing septations within. Lung window corroborates the findings.

Discussion

Tuberculosis in the liver is usually a/w pulmonary (spread via hepatic artery) or gastrointestinal tract (via portal vein) tuberculosis. It may present as:

- Miliary pattern with tiny hypodense granulomas on CT or echogenic liver on sonography.
- *Tuberculomas*: Hypoechoic/dense lesion (caseous necrosis) with minimal peripheral enhancement (granulation tissue).
- *Abscess*: Irregular, thick-walled heterogeneously enhancing hypoechoic/dense complex lesion with associated coalescent small hypoechoic/dense tubercles.
- Biliary tract involvement appears as stricture formation, duct wall thickening, and dilatation.

Discussed in the first chapter.

Management

Antitubercular therapy +/– abscess drainage.

Case 158 Disseminated Tuberculosis

A 38-year-old patient with systemic symptoms and weight loss (Figure 9.4).

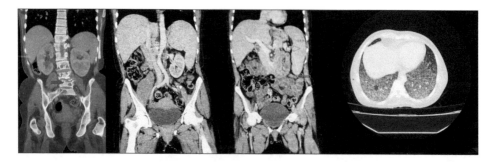

Figure 9.4 CECT abdomen depicts bony destruction (solid arrows), bilateral psoas abscesses with calcific foci (arrowhead) in the left psoas, splenomegaly, and miliary lung pattern (star) in disseminated tuberculosis.

Discussion

Disseminated tuberculosis refers to the concomitant involvement of at least two non-contiguous body parts or infection of the blood, bone marrow, or liver due to hematogenous spread of Mycobacterium tuberculosis. It can affect any body part.

Miliary tuberculosis (millet seed-sized (1–2 mm) tuberculous foci) is a potentially fatal form of disseminated disease, especially in immunosuppressed patients. The thoracic and lumbar vertebrae are primarily affected by tuberculous spondylitis (Pott's disease), which causes widespread bone destruction, compressive fracture, and extension to soft tissues, including epidural and paraspinal psoas "cold" abscess. Calcific foci in the psoas abscess are pathognomic of TB. CT, and MRI better delineate the presence and extent of disease. Abscesses are hypodense on CT, hypointense on T1WI, and hyperintense on T2WI with rim enhancement.

Differentials

- Pyogenic infections (rapidly progressive/acute)
- Metastasis (preserved disc space)

Management

- Antituberculous therapy
- Symptomatic management

Case 159 Sclerosing Encapsulated Peritonitis (Abdominal Cocoon)

A 25-year-old female presented with vomiting and abdominal pain (Figure 9.5).

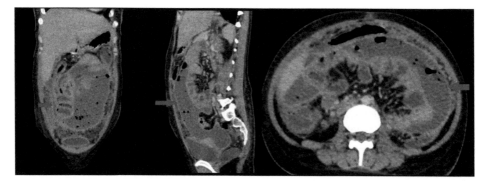

Figure 9.5 CT enterography depicts a central congregation of bowel loops encased by a peripherally enhancing, thickened peritoneum forming a sac-like structure (abdominal cocoon arrow) around the bowel loops with thick hypodense collection and multiple post-procedural air foci within. Omental caking, mesenteric fat stranding, and IC junction thickening are noted in a known case of tuberculosis.

Discussion

Encapsulating peritoneal sclerosis (EPS), also termed abdominal cocoon, is an uncommon though alarming entity leading to thickened fibro-collagen membrane encasing the bowel loops and recurring bowel obstruction incidents. Sonography depicts the central clustering of bowel loops adherent to the anterior abdominal wall, interloop ascites, peristaltic changes, LAP, and membrane encapsulation. CECT corroborates the findings with a smoothly thickened enhancing peritoneal sac (cocoon) encasing the congregation of intestines centrally.

Differentials

- Peritonitis due to peritoneal dialysis (shift to hemodialysis and total parenteral nutrition), previous abdominal surgery, sclerosing serositis due to long-term use of practolol (selective beta-1 blocker).

- Peritoneal carcinomatosis (nodular irregular thickening a/w primary ovarian/gastric cancer and nodules in the omentum and the serosal surfaces).

- Internal hernia (cocoon in EPS will displace the mesenteric vessels posteriorly).

- Congenital peritoneal encapsulation (thin peritoneal membrane around the intestines, discovered incidentally during surgery).

Management

Surgery on cases complicated with ischemia/obstruction, adhesiolysis, and cocoon dissection.

Case 160 Prostatic Tubercular Abscess

A 19-year-old male with known TB (Figure 9.6).

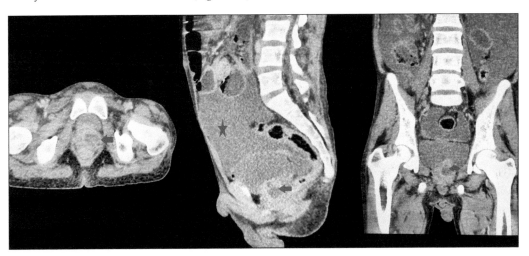

Figure 9.6 CECT abdomen shows a mildly enlarged prostate with a peripherally enhancing hypoattenuating lesion on the left side of the prostate along with gross ascites.

Discussion

Granulomatous prostatitis is usually asymptomatic and spreads via a hematogenous route in a patient with pulmonary or renal tuberculosis. Laboratory findings include raised PSA (prostate-specific-antigen) and sterile pyuria. On rectal examination, a prostatic tuberculous abscess is depicted as a nodular or enlarged prostate. Imaging reveals an irregular hypoechoic/attenuated area with peripheral enhancement and restricted diffusion and may show a watermelon sign. Transrectal sonography/MRI reveals the lesion in the peripheral zone. Perirectal extension may occur in large abscesses. Dystrophic calcifications may be seen in chronic cases. Urethral involvement with stricture formation, urethroperineal fistula (watering can perineum), or ulcerative penile lesion may occur in a few cases (Table 9.1).

Differentials

- Bacterial prostatic abscess (leukocytes, fever, and pain)

- Infected prostatic utricle cyst/retention cyst

- Cystic degeneration of BPH

- TURP (transurethral resection of the prostate) defect

- Prostatic adenocarcinoma (more enhancement and more restriction on DWI)

Management

Antitubercular therapy with follow-up

Case 161 Bilateral Tubercular Tubo-Ovarian Abscesses

A 30-year-old female with fever and pelvic pain (Figure 9.7).

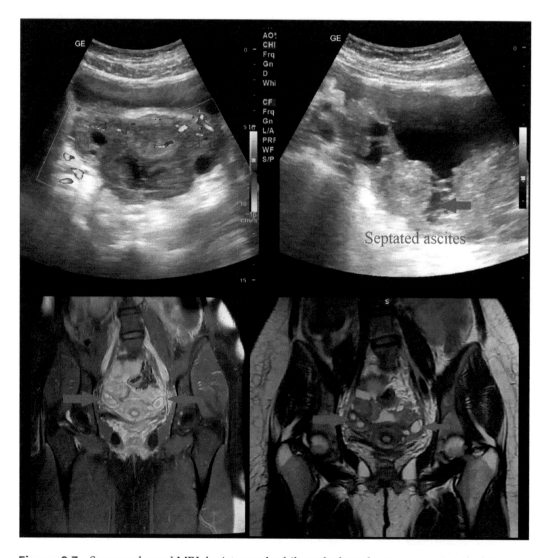

Figure 9.7 Sonography and MRI depict complex bilateral adnexal masses encasing the lateral and posterior walls of the uterus and extending into the pouch of Douglas. Bilateral ovaries are not seen separate from the mass. Moderate ascites with thick septations in the pelvic cavity. Peritoneal thickening in the pelvic cavity and inflamed echogenic omental fat.

Discussion

Tubo-ovarian abscess, grave sequelae of pelvic inflammatory disease, occurs due to the spread of mycobacterial infection from the lower genital tract, initially involving fallopian tubes and then to ovaries along with the uterus and peritoneal space. Patients may present with altered menstrual cycle, amenorrhoea, and infertility. Sonography reveals complex solid-cystic heteroechoic adnexal lesions with increased vascularity. Tuberculosis may involve peritoneal and omental thickening, fat stranding, and septated ascites. Lesions are hypointense on T1WI and heterogeneously hyperintense on T2WI with alteration in signal intensity depending on the viscosity and continents of the abscess (discussed in Table 9.1 and Chapter 5).

Differential Diagnosis

- Ovarian malignancy with peritoneal carcinomatosis
- Actinomycosis/Bacteroides infection
- Ovarian metastasis

Management

Antitubercular therapy

Case 162 Pott's Spine with Psoas Abscess

A 40-year-old male known tubercular patient with fever, backache, and weight loss (Figure 9.8).

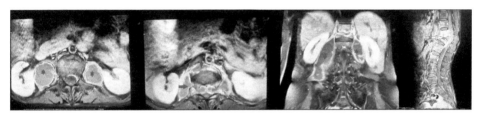

Figure 9.8 MRI of another patient revealed vertebral destruction with pre and paravertebral abscesses—bilateral psoas (star) and anterior epidural abscesses (solid arrow) with vertebral body destruction.

Discussion

Pott's disease/tuberculous spondylitis, the contiguous involvement of multiple vertebral bodies, is the common form of extrapulmonary tuberculosis with slow progression. Patients present with long-standing backache, which may get complicated as paraplegia due to cord compression and kyphotic deformity. CT depicts the varying patterns of destruction (fragmentary, osteolytic, sclerotic, and subperiosteal) with multiloculated cystic paraspinal abscesses that appear mixed signal intensity on T1- and T2WI with heterogeneous enhancement depending on the viscosity and contents. These abscesses tend to extend along the tissue planes and epidural space. Calcification within abscess is pathognomic of tuberculosis.

Patterns of vertebral body involvement are discussed (Table 9.2).

Table 9.2: Patterns of Vertebral Body Involvement in TB

Paradiscal	Blurred para discal margins Joint space narrowing Anterior wedging/collapse (kyphotic deformity)
Anterior sub ligamentous (subperiosteal)	Fusiform appearance with anterior scalloping (aneurysmal) Disc space preserved
Central	Destruction and ballooning of vertebral bodies Concentric collapse (vertebra plana) Disc space preserved
Posterior/neural arch	Posterior elements destruction Erosion of adjacent ribs Sparing of intervertebral discs Large paraspinal mass

Differentials

- Pyogenic/fungal spondylitis (acute and relatively fast progression of symptoms; disc involvement even in early stages, 1–2 vertebral bodies involvement, irregular rim enhancement)
- Metastasis

Management

- Antitubercular therapy,
- Percutaneous drainage or surgical debridement

ROLE OF AI IN ABDOMINOPELVIC RADIOLOGY

INTRODUCTION

The role of artificial intelligence (AI) in abdominopelvic radiology is transformative, offering enhanced efficiency, accuracy, and potential for early diagnosis. Here are vital aspects:

Automated Image Analysis: AI algorithms can swiftly analyze vast abdominopelvic images, automating routine tasks like organ segmentation and lesion detection.

a. Segmentation involves delineating the boundary of an organ or lesion of interest in radiologic images. It gives us information about the volume, shape, and densities of a target organ or lesion, which can be utilized to gauge its severity or make medical diagnoses. Multiorgan segmentation models can segment multiple organs simultaneously with comparable levels of accuracy. More intricate substructures, like the hepatic vasculature, the Couinaud liver segments, the anatomy of the biliary tree, and the prostate zonal anatomy, are now the focus of the segmentation work.

b. Lesion detection involves finding the precise location of an abnormality in the image. Early detection of tumors or lesions increases the chances of successful treatment.

c. Differentiating the necrotic active components of the liver tumor to determine the exact tumor burden.

d. Transfer learning radiomics models, using elastography can classify liver fibrosis better.

e. Promising outcomes have been shown in detecting calcific plaques in the aorta, muscle density, ratio of visceral/subcutaneous fat, liver attenuation, vertebral density, and segmenting other non-tumoral disease entities, such as urinary calculi, hemo/pneumoperitoneum, and colonic polyps.

Workflow Optimization: By streamlining repetitive processes, AI allows radiologists to focus on complex cases, improving workflow efficiency. It can also prioritize workflow in the automated detection of incidental findings, including free fluid, fat stranding, vertebral body fractures, and pulmonary embolism.

Quantitative Analysis: AI aids in the quantitative analysis of imaging data, providing precise measurements and assessments for a more comprehensive diagnostic approach.

- Volume assessment of the liver segments prior to surgical removal for donation or liver transplantation.
- Assessment of the total kidney volume in patients with polycystic kidney disease.
- Evaluating liver fat and iron concentration.

Clinical Decision Support Systems: AI offers additional insights and recommendations based on data analysis, literature, and established protocols.

Differential Diagnosis: AI algorithms can help generate potential diagnoses, providing valuable guidance to radiologists in complex cases. Hepatic, pancreatic, renal, adrenal, prostate, ovarian, and cervical neoplasms can be classified as benign or malignant. It helps in differentiating:

- Lipid-poor renal AML from RCC in CT
- HCC from intrahepatic cholangiocarcinoma in CT
- Stromal benign prostatic hyperplasia from transitional zone prostate cancer
- Benign borderline ovarian tumors from malignant ovarian tumors

Personalized Medicine

Combining radiomics features with machine learning techniques makes it possible to predict clinical outcomes, identify novel image biomarkers for well-known diseases, forecast specific gene expression, identify early recurrence, and predict treatment response or overall survival in various cancers. Models can indicate intraoperative blood loss in placenta previa, hepatic encephalopathy in cirrhotic liver CT, and future occurrences of gastro-esophageal variceal bleeding. Hence, AI applications can contribute to personalized treatment plans by analyzing patient-specific data and selecting the most effective interventions.

Image Reconstruction

- *Noise Reduction*: AI algorithms can enhance image quality by reducing scan noise, leading to more explicit and detailed abdominopelvic images.

- *Artifact Correction*: AI techniques can correct imaging artifacts, ensuring more accurate and reliable diagnostic information.

- The software enables lower radiation doses to be used in CT exams.

Research and Data Analysis

- *Big Data Utilization*: AI facilitates the analysis of large datasets, enabling radiologists and researchers to identify patterns and correlations that may not be apparent through traditional methods.

- *Predictive Analytics*: AI contributes to predictive modeling, helping anticipate disease progression and patient outcomes. Progressive loss of muscle bulk, function, or quality has been shown to predict overall unfavorable and progression-free survival in cancer patients.

Training and Education

AI systems can continuously learn from new data, ensuring they stay updated with the latest medical knowledge and diagnostic trends.

Challenges of Artificial Intelligence Application and Future Works

1. The abdominopelvic region contains various organs with complicated architecture, anatomical variability, proximity to other organs, and constant mobility, making segmentation and detection difficult.

2. Most research uses a meticulously gathered dataset to focus on a particular organ, a single phase or sequence, and a specific disease state. However, the real-world work requires several diagnoses on multiple organs, and further research on universal multitask algorithms is needed.

3. Furthermore, the real-world dataset may present a more comprehensive range of disorders and a substantially lower disease prevalence. Therefore, more studies on larger imaging datasets with outside validation are required.

4. When interpreting the findings of the abdominal AI scans, caution is advisable as the algorithm's accuracy depends on the trained dataset, which further depends on the imaging modality, scanner types, and protocol used to select the gold standard. More clinical validation is needed for AI to help radiologists and clinicians.

Future Directives

The technology for robot-assisted endoscopic equipment has evolved significantly. These robots could undertake a surgical procedure or automatically obtain a biopsy sample from a lesion if they collaborate with an intelligent system that detects lesions via ultrasound, obviating the complexities of endoscopic and surgical procedures.

SUGGESTED READINGS

Akhan, O., & Pringot, J. Imaging of abdominal tuberculosis. *Eur Radiol.* 2002;12(2):312–323. doi: 10.1007/s003300100994.

Burrill, J., Williams, C. J., Bain, G., Conder, G., Hine, A. L. & Misra, R. R. Tuberculosis: A radiologic review. *Radiographics* 2007;27:5, 1255–1273.

Chang, K. P., Lin, S. H., & Chu, Y. W. Artificial intelligence in gastrointestinal radiology: A review with special focus on recent development of magnetic resonance and computed tomography. *Artif Intell Gastroenterol.* 2021;2(2):27–41. doi: 10.35712/aig.v2.i2.27.

da Rocha, E. L. et al. Abdominal tuberculosis: A radiological review with emphasis on computed tomography and magnetic resonance imaging findings. *Radiol Bras.* 2015;48(3):181–191. doi: 10.1590/0100-3984.2013.1801.

European Society of Radiology (ESR). What the radiologist should know about artificial intelligence - an ESR white paper. *Insights Imaging* 2019;10:44. doi: 10.1186/s13244-019-0738-2.

10 Image-Based Multiple Choice Questions

Q1. What is the diagnosis in a patient with an enlarged left kidney with multiple low-attenuation peripherally enhancing masses replacing the renal parenchyma? (Figure 10.1)

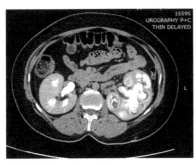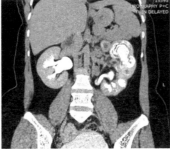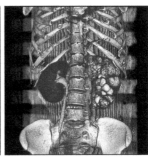

Figure 10.1

    a. Staghorn calculus

    b. Xanthogranulomatous pyelonephritis

    c. Lymphoma

    d. Page kidney

Q2. In Figure 10.2, the main cause of this condition with respiratory distress is

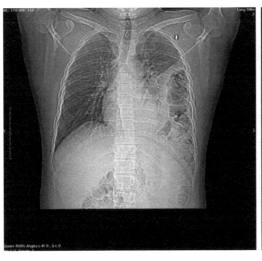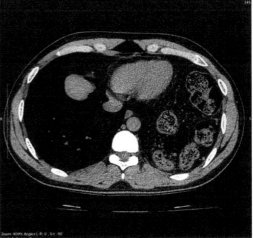

Figure 10.2

    a. Reduced clearance of fluid from the lungs

    b. Insufficient surfactant production

    c. Defective closure of the pleuroperitoneal canal

    d. Meconium aspiration

DOI: 10.1201/9781003452034-10

Q3. Diagnosis in this patient (Figure 10.3)

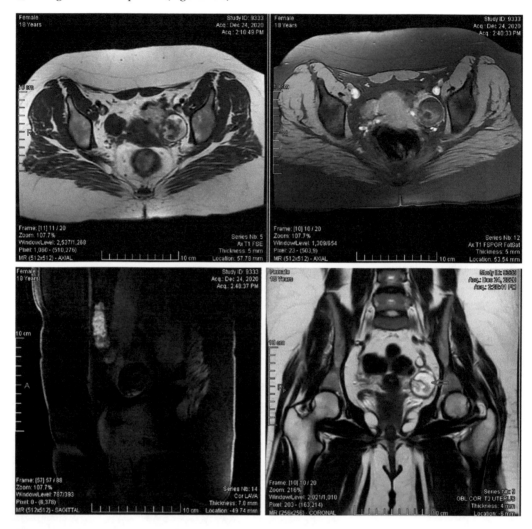

Figure 10.3

   a. Ovarian dermoid

   b. Sacrococcygeal teratoma

   c. Endometriosis

   d. Ruptured ectopic pregnancy

Q4. Diagnosis (Figure 10.4)

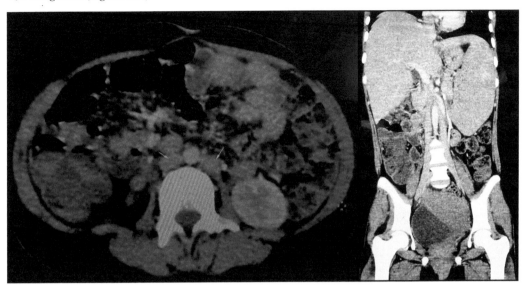

Figure 10.4

a. Circumaortic left renal vein

b. Duplicated vena cava

c. Duplicated aorta

d. Persistent gonadal vessels

Q5. Diagnosis (Figure 10.5)

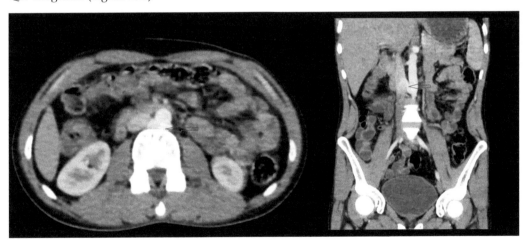

Figure 10.5

a. Retroaortic left renal vein

b. Duplicated aorta

c. Persistent right gonadal vein

d. Hemizygous continuation of IVC

Q6. Differentials may include all of the following except (Figure 10.6)

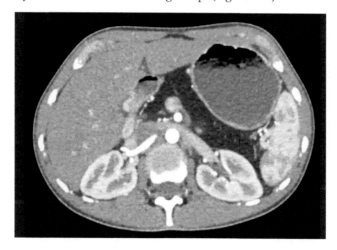

Figure 10.6

    a. Cystic fibrosis

    b. Schwachmann–Diamond syndrome

    c. Aging

    d. Agenesis

Q7. Diagnosis (Figure 10.7)

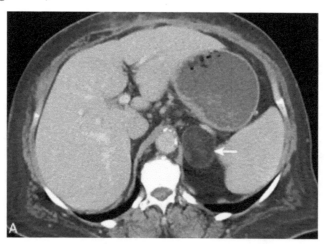

Figure 10.7

    a. Adrenal adenoma

    b. Myelolipoma

    c. Pheochromocytoma

    d. Complex renal cyst

Q8. Diagnosis (Figure 10.8)

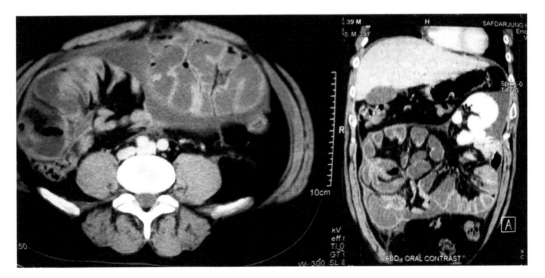

Figure 10.8

a. Encapsulating peritoneal sclerosis

b. Ovarian malignancy

c. Vascular anomaly

d. Trauma

Q9. Diagnosis (Figure 10.9)

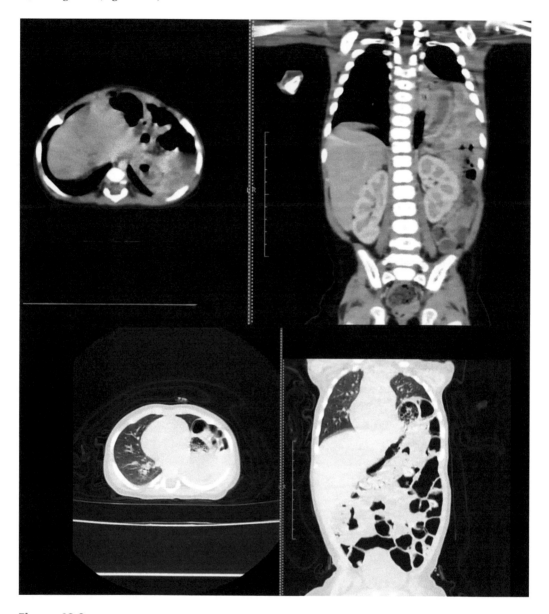

Figure 10.9

    a.   Morgagni's hernia

    b.   Traumatic rupture of diaphragm

    c.   Bochdalek's hernia

    d.   Mallory-Weis syndrome

Q10. Characteristic findings include (Figure 10.10)

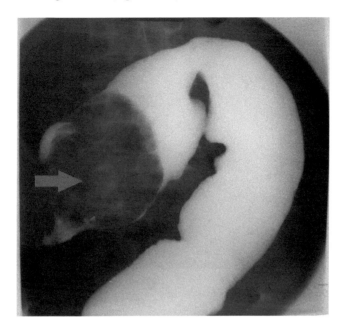

Figure 10.10

    a. Degeneration of vitelline duct

    b. Rigler triad

    c. Bowel within bowel appearance

    d. Thumbprinting

Q11. Characteristic signs include all except (Figure 10.11)

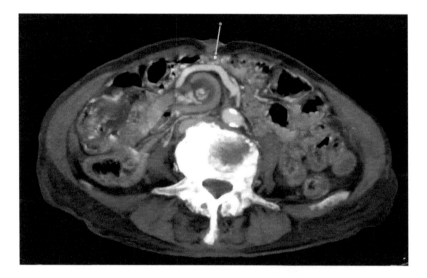

Figure 10.11

    a. Whirlpool sign

    b. Malrotated bowel

    c. Corkscrew sign

    d. Antral nipple sign

Q12. Procedure done in this image (Figure 10.12)

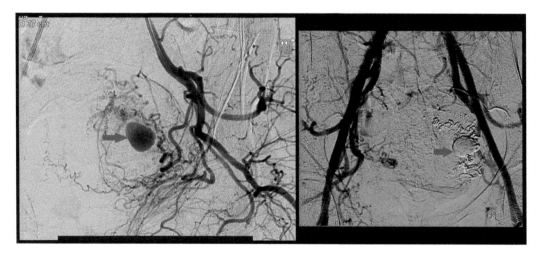

Figure 10.12

    a. GDA aneurysm coiling

    b. Uterine artery embolization

    c. SMA coiling

    d. RAS stenting

Q13. Diagnosis of this non-enhancing lesion in a patient with history of trauma (Figure 10.13)

    a. Pseudopancreatic cyst

    b. Adrenal cyst

    c. Biliary cyst

    d. Mesenteric cyst

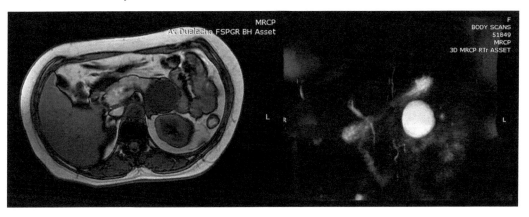

Figure 10.13

Q14. Diagnosis of the non-enhancing lesion (arrow) in a patient with history of fever and travel (Figure 10.14)

    a. Metastasis

    b. Hepatocellular carcinoma

    c. Abscess

    d. Simple liver cyst

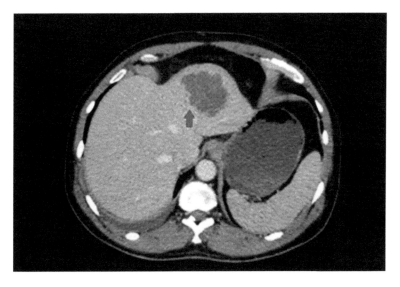

Figure 10.14

Q15. A 61-year-old patient presented with abdominal pain, fever, not passing stool for 10 days along with neutrophilia (Figure 10.15)

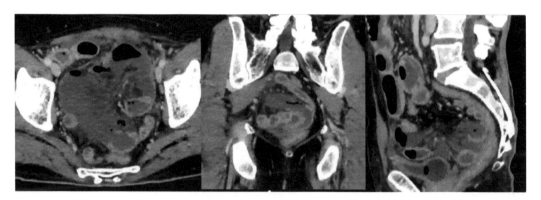

Figure 10.15

    a. Appendicitis

    b. Perforation peritonitis

    c. Torsion

    d. Adenocarcinoma.

Q16. Characteristics features in this 64-year-old patient include all except (Figure 10.16)

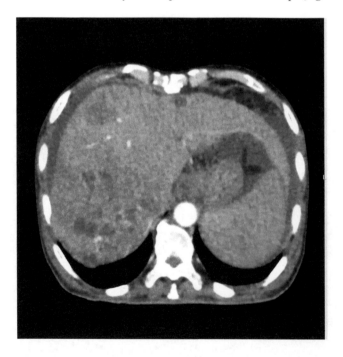

Figure 10.16

    a. Early washout in the lesion in the portovenous phase

    b. Tumoral thrombus

   c.   Centripetal fill-in

   d.   Neoangiogenesis

Q17. Metastasis from which primary malignancy (Figure 10.17)

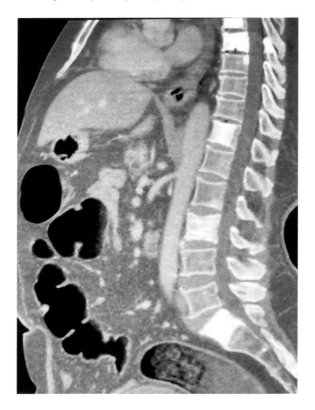

Figure 10.17

   a.   Renal cell carcinoma

   b.   Hepatocellular carcinoma

   c.   Thyroid carcinoma

   d.   Prostate carcinoma

Q18. Diagnosis in this patient with mobile echogenic lesion in the bladder (Figure 10.18)

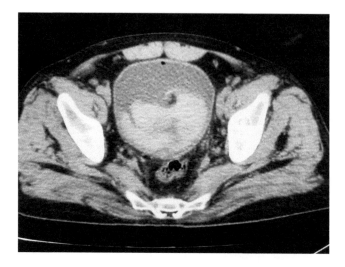

Figure 10.18

    a. Transitional cell carcinoma

    b. Papillary carcinoma

    c. Hematoma

    d. Jackstone calculus

Q19. Diagnosis in Figure 10.19

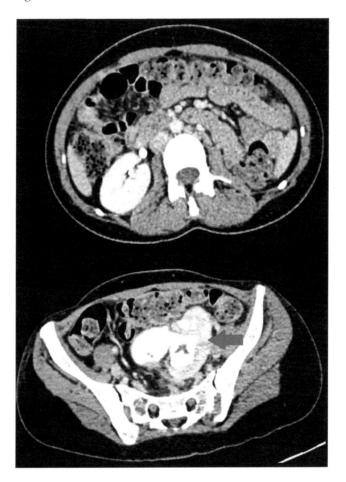

Figure 10.19

    a. Pancake kidney

    b. Horseshoe kidney

    c. Ectopic kidney

    d. Duplex kidney

Q20. All of the following is true about the image (Figure 10.20) except

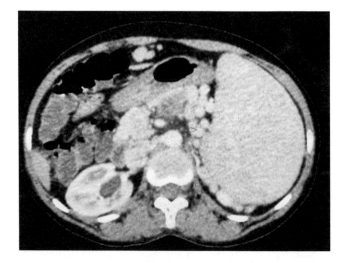

Figure 10.20

    a. Splenomegaly

    b. Recanalized paraumbilical vein

    c. Dilated superior mesenteric artery

    d. Low flow velocity in the portal vein

Q21. Diagnosis in Figure 10.21

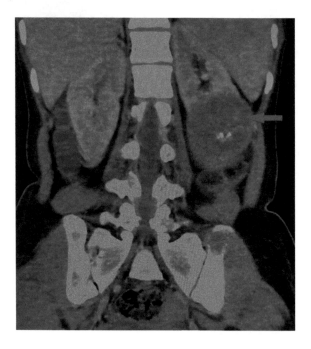

Figure 10.21

a. Birt Hogg Dube syndrome

b. Renal cell carcinoma

c. Angiomyolipoma

d. Nephroblastoma

Q22. All of the following are true for Figure 10.22 except

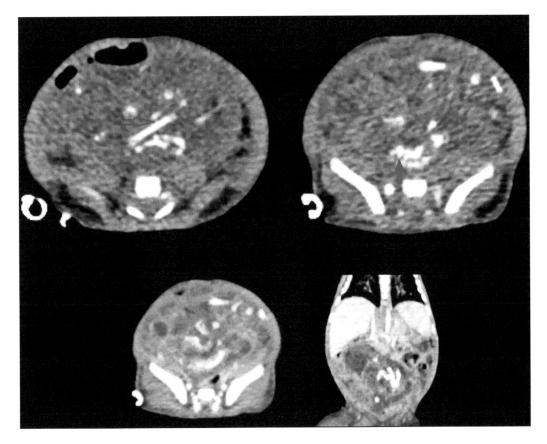

Figure 10.22

a. Non-viable fetus becomes encased in a regularly developing fetus

b. Usually during a monochorionic diamniotic pregnancy

c. Differential is intra-abdominal teratoma

d. Diagnosis is hepatoblastoma

Q23. Arrow in the Figure 10.23 suggests

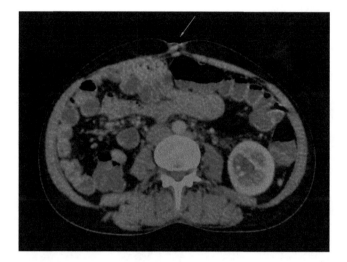

Figure 10.23

  a. Abscess
  b. Portal hypertension
  c. Urachal fistula
  d. Sebaceous cyst

Q24. Diagnosis in Figure 10.24

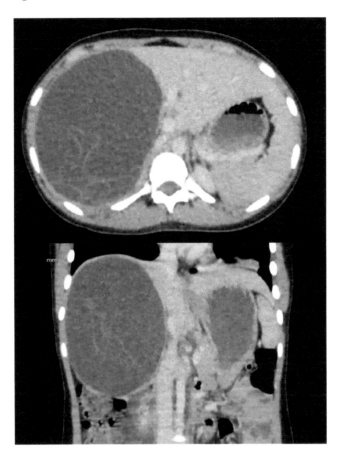

Figure 10.24

    a. Pyogenic abscess

    b. Biliary cystadenoma

    c. Hydatid cyst

    d. Cystic HCC

Q25. Discuss the diagnosis (Figure 10.25)

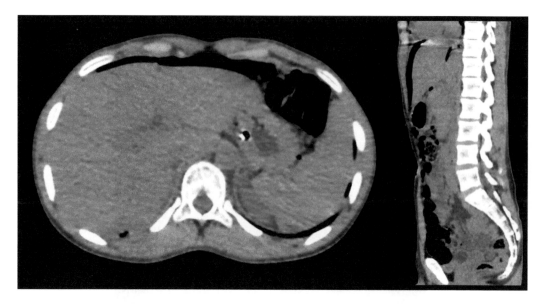

Figure 10.25

    a. Chiladiti syndrome

    b. Pneumoperitoneum

    c. Abscess

    d. Metastasis

Q26. Diagnosis (Figure 10.26)

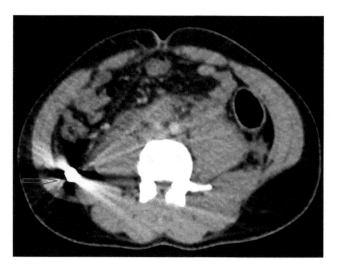

Figure 10.26

    a. Truncation artifacts

    b. Partial volume averaging

    c. Beam hardening artifacts

    d. Zebra artifacts

Q27. Diagnosis (Figure 10.27)

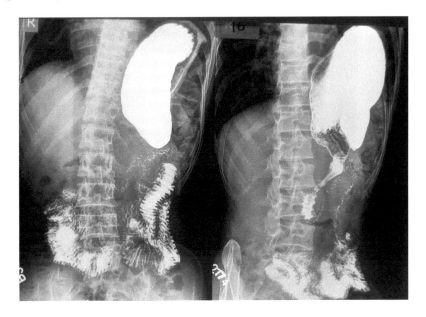

Figure 10.27

    a. Post-operative status

    b. Ladd bands

    c. Diabetic gastroparesis

    d. Twisting of the stomach on its mesentery

Q28. Characteristic findings include (Figure 10.28)

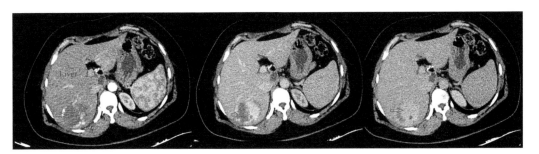

Figure 10.28

    a. Early washout in the lesion in the portovenous phase

    b. Tumoral thrombus

    c. Centripetal fill-in

    d. Neoangiogenesis

Q29. Which of the following is true in a patient with recent biliary instrumentation? (Figure 10.29)

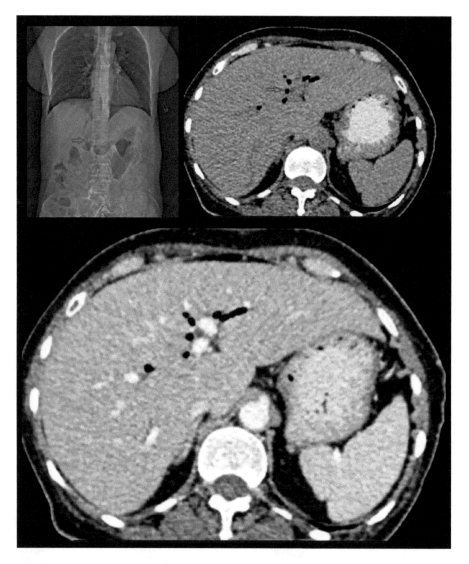

Figure 10.29

    a. Gas in the biliary radicles

    b. Gas in the portal venous system

    c. Peripheral linear lucencies

    d. Scattered fat globules

Q30. All of the following are true for Figure 10.30 except

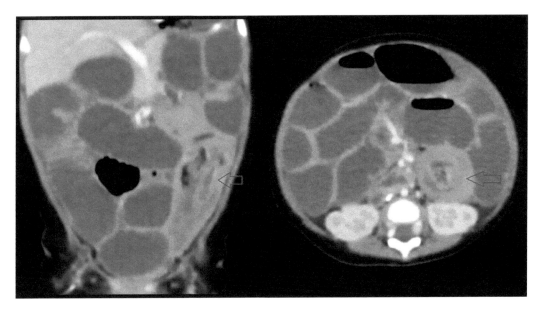

Figure 10.30

    a. Intussusceptum is the prolapsing part of the bowel

    b. Intussusceptum is the receiving end of the bowel

    c. Intussuscipiens is the distal segment of bowel receiving the intussusceptum

    d. Incorporation of mesentery results in comprise of venous return and edema

Answers to Multiple Choice Questions

1. B
2. C (diagnosis is congenital diaphragmatic hernia)
3. A
4. B
5. A
6. D (fatty replacement of pancreas-strands of acinar tissue and ductal structures visible)
7. A
8. A
9. C
10. C
11. D
12. B
13. A
14. C
15. B
16. C
17. D
18. C
19. C (Ectopic and mal-rotated left kidney)
20. C
21. B
22. D (fetus-in-fetu with femur as an open arrow and spine as a solid arrow)
23. B
24. C
25. B
26. C (metallic streak artifacts due to bullet)
27. D
28. C
29. A (Gas within the biliary tree tends to be more central, whereas gas within the portal venous system tends to be peripheral)
30. B

Index

Note: **Bold** page numbers refer to tables and *italic* page numbers refer to figures.

T - #0274 - 160425 - C256 - 254/178/12 - PB - 9781032587745 - Gloss Lamination